The Art & Science of Manicuring

By Alice R. Cimaglia

Milady Publishing Company
(A Division of Delmar Publishers Inc.)
220 White Plains Road, Tarrytown, NY 10591

Copyright © 1982, 1986

Published by
Milady Publishing Company
(A Division of Delmar Publishers Inc.)
Tarrytown, NY 10591

Printed in the United States of America

ISBN 0-87350-409-7

10 9 8 7 6 5 4

FOREWORD

The information in this book on the art and science of manicuring has been completely revised and brought up to date.

The science of manicuring consists of knowledge, which is factual and systematic. The art of manicuring, which involves doing, varies with the technique employed by each individual manicurist.

The manicurist will find the basic techniques described in this book flexible and adaptable to the routine being followed in beauty salons and barber-styling shops.

To derive the most benefit from this book, demonstration and practice should accompany theoretical study.

Success in manicuring depends on study, hard work and perseverance.

The Author

Contents

Salon Conduct

Manicuring *(man'i-kyur-ing)* **as a career** offers many opportunities and rewards to those students who have acquired thorough training and have developed an attractive appearance and a charming personality.

Salon conduct embraces the attitude and behavior of the manicurist and reveals itself in the personal dealings with employer, clients and associates. The manicurist who is considerate of other people's thoughts and feelings will have no difficulty in maintaining a high standard of salon conduct. To keep on improving his or her shop conduct, the manicurist should strive to cultivate the habits of good character, vibrant health and careful grooming.

Success in manicuring can be acquired by observing the rules of salon conduct. The daily practice of these rules will help the manicurist achieve the ambition of contentment on the job, personal advancement, and happiness. By gaining a favorable reputation, the manicurist will become eligible for higher paying positions. To reach these goals, *obey the following rules of salon conduct:*

1. **Be punctual.** Get to work on time and be prompt with all appointments.
2. **Be courteous.** Have a sunny disposition. Be cheerful, be friendly and be dignified to clients.
3. **Perform all tasks** willingly and efficiently.
4. **Be clean,** neat, attractive and orderly in your work.
5. **Learn to talk** clearly and intelligently and listen attentively when engaging in a conversation.
6. **Show respect** and consideration to clients, co-workers and employer or manager.
7. **Be honest** with your clients.
8. **Be loyal** to your employer or manager.
9. **Avoid gossip** and loud talk in the presence of clients.
10. **Lift your feet** when walking—do not shuffle.

To Be Successful...

To be successful you must learn to do the little things that are appreciated by clients and make them want to come back to see you again and again.

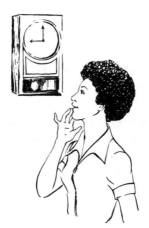

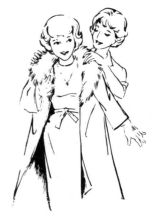

Be punctual.
Get to work on time and you won't miss any clients.

Tardiness never pays.

Be courteous.
Treat people with the same kindness you would want to be treated, and everyone will like you.

Discourtesy is inexcusable.

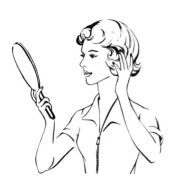

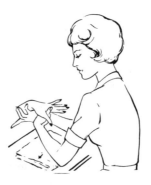

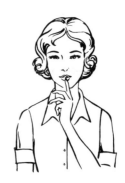

Be neat, clean and attractive.

Be good to look at, and clients will admire you.

Slovenliness in dress or hygiene is offensive.

Be gentle. You will be remembered for this valued characteristic.

Harsh, rough treatment chases clients away.

Mind your own business. Clients will trust you.

Gab and they won't like you.

Professional Ethics

Professional ethics deal with the proper conduct and business dealings of the manicurist in relation to his or her employer, clients and co-workers. The essential considerations in professional ethics are honesty, fairness, courtesy and respect for the feelings and rights of others. The ethical manicurist always gives the best possible service to clients, keeping in mind their desires, needs and welfare.

To build public confidence and retain a good following, the individual manicurist should live up to these rules of ethics:

1. Acquire a thorough knowledge of manicuring.
2. Believe in your chosen profession sincerely and practice it conscientiously.
3. Keep your word and fulfill all your obligations.
4. Obey all provisions of the state laws covering manicuring.
5. Cherish a good reputation and set an example of good conduct and behavior.
6. Treat all clients fairly; do not show any favoritism.
7. Be loyal to your employer and associates.

Ethics are violated by resorting to questionable practices, extravagant claims and unfulfilled promises which cast an unfavorable light on cosmetology in general and the individual manicurist in particular.

The Successful Manicurist

1. Should be thoroughly proficient in work, both practically and scientifically.
2. Should be ever mindful of hygienic habits, being extremely careful to avoid having bad breath and body odor.
3. Should adopt a cordial manner in greeting clients and in speaking over the telephone.
4. Should remember that first impressions are lasting, and to that end should cultivate charm and personality.
5. Should plan each day's schedule with proper thought.

6. Should arrange appointments carefully so that long waits will be avoided.

7. Should avoid entering into discussions with the client concerning personal problems.

8. Should handle clients tactfully, and endeavor to maintain an even temperament.

9. Should adopt a manner of approach that will impress confidence in the client.

10. Should avoid the offensive practice of chewing or smoking in the presence of clients.

11. Should never speak disparagingly of the service rendered by other manicurists, cosmetologists, or salons.

12. Should do the little things appreciated by clients.

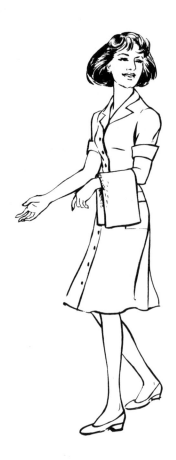

Introduction to Manicuring

Women through the ages have practiced manicuring in order to keep their hands beautiful. Along with the changes in styles of dress and hair fashions, the standard of beautiful hands has also changed. The ideal hand of our modern generation is one that is long and slender, with tapering fingers, skin that is soft and smooth, and fingernails that are carefully manicured to enhance the beauty of the hands.

Manicuring is not limited to the hands of women. More and more men request the services of a manicurist when they visit the barber-styling shop or full service salons.

The word *manicuring* is derived from the Latin-*manus* (hand) and *cura* (care), meaning care of the hands and nails. The purpose of a manicure therefore, is to cleanse the hands and nails and improve their appearance.

A manicurist is entrusted with the beauty care of a client's hands. To be adept in the art of manicuring requires not only thorough preparation but continual practice to develop skill.

A good manicurist must also realize the importance of sanitation for the protection of his or her own health as well as that of the client. It is also necessary to know the science of bacteriology in order to understand how disease is transmitted and to be able to recognize those that are contagious.

Through knowledge and training, a manicurist can become aware of the client's physical condition. Clammy hands, for example, often signify nervousness, and large knuckles may indicate rheumatism.

Hands are a dramatic form of expression. They are also a great give-away of age. It is, therefore, part of the manicurist's duty to keep the muscles taut and the flesh firm. This will be achieved by exercise and treatment.

By diligent study and constant practice, you can become a successful manicurist. *You will have a profession with a future!*

A Well-Groomed Manicurist

The manicurist's care for personal appearance is the best advertisement to a client.

To keep your appearance at its best, give daily attention to all the important details which make for a clean, neat and charming personality.

Daily Bath and Deodorant

Keep the body fresh by having a daily shower or bath and by using an underarm deodorant.

Teeth and Breath
Clean and brush the teeth regularly.
Use mouthwash to sweeten the breath.

Hairstyle
Keep the hair clean, lustrous and in place
and have an attractive and practical
hairstyle at all times.

Clothes
Wear a uniform that is spotlessly clean,
neat and properly fitted.

Facial Makeup
Use the correct cosmetics to match your
skin tones. Have a fresh, flawless
complexion, sparking eyes, well-shaped
eyebrows and lips.

Hands and Nails
Keep your hands clean and smooth and
your nails well-manicured.

Jewelry
Avoid gaudy jewelry, long, hanging
necklaces, and large bracelets.

Shoes and Stockings
Wear low-heeled shoes that are well-fitted
and sensibly styled. Keep the shoes shined
and in good condition. Wear clean hose.
Watch out for hosiery runs and wrinkles.

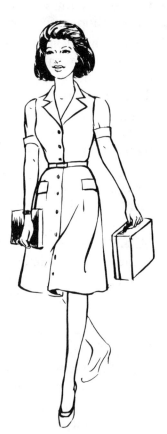

*A Well-Groomed
Manicurist*

Hygiene and Personality
Personal Hygiene

Hygiene *(hy'jeen)* is that science that deals with the prevention of disease and the preservation and improvement of health. It includes personal hygiene and public hygiene.

Personal hygiene concerns the intelligent care exercised by the individual to preserve health through following the rules of healthful living.

Public hygiene or **sanitation** refers to the measures used by governmental agencies to preserve and promote public health, such as provisions for a pure supply of air, food and water, the proper disposal of sewage and the control of disease.

To preserve public health, any person suffering from an infectious *(in-fek'shus)* or contagious *(kon-tay'jus)* disease in any communicable *(kuh-myun'i-ka-bl)* form should not be allowed to work in a beauty salon.

Beauty problems are also **health problems.** An improvement in health reflects itself in a better complexion, a fine textured skin, sparkling eyes and luxuriant hair. The complexion is the outward expression of inner health. A dull, sallow complexion is indicative of a sluggish circulation, lack of fresh air and irregular elimination of waste products from the body. Therefore, to improve your health and beauty, you must follow hygienic rules of living.

A faulty diet is one of the basic causes of poor health. Avoid such poor eating habits as:

1. Not eating enough of the right kinds of food, which may lead to loss of weight, lowered resistance, or nutritional diseases.
2. Overeating, which overworks the digestive system and organs of elimination.

Eating well-balanced meals at regular intervals and drinking a sufficient quantity of water will keep the digestive system functioning properly and produce better elimination.

Exercise and recreation in the form of walking, dancing, sports and gym activities develop muscles, besides keeping the body fit. Among the benefits resulting from regular and nonstrenuous exercise are an improvement in nutrition and blood circulation. The body is supplied with more life-giving oxygen due to the increased action of the lungs. Moderate amounts of sunshine add vigor and help to supply the body with essential vitamin D.

Fatigue or tiredness, resulting from work, exercise, mental effort or the strain caused by hurry and worry, should always be followed by a period of rest or relaxation. Overexertion and lack of rest tend to drain the body of its vitality. Therefore, an adequate amount of sleep, about seven hours, is necessary. This allows the body to recover from the fatigue of the day's activities and replenish itself with renewed energy for the next day's work.

Personal Cleanliness

Personal cleanliness is an important hygienic *(hy-jee-en' ik)* habit. The manicurist must observe cleanliness in the following ways:

1. Keep body clean by having a daily bath or shower.
2. Avoid offensive body odors by using a deodorant regularly.
3. Keep teeth and gums in good condition, and the breath sweet by brushing the teeth twice daily.
4. Have periodic examinations of the teeth by a good dentist. All decayed teeth should be filled or removed.
5. Treat bad or offensive breath by gargling with a good antiseptic.
6. Wear clean stockings, clean undergarments and a clean uniform.
7. Wash hands before and after serving each client, and after visiting the toilet.
8. Avoid the use in common of towels, drinking cups, powder puffs, hairpins, hairbrushes and combs.

To maintain good health, observe the following rules:

1. Have proper housing and ventilation.
2. Have plenty of outdoor recreation and exercise.
3. Breathe deeply, expanding the lungs as much as possible.
4. Eat only what is actually desired; do not overeat, and chew food thoroughly.
5. Drink sufficient water each day.
6. Stand, sit and walk erectly.
7. Have regular physical examinations to check the health of the body.

Posture for Sitting

Maintaining the correct sitting posture at the manicure table helps to avoid body fatigue and backstrain. As a manicurist, you will be in a sitting position most of the day. Try to sit with the lower back near the back of the chair, leaning slightly foreward while working on your client. If a stool is used, place your entire body weight on the stool.

To prevent any armstrain, adjust the client's chair far enough away from the manicure table to allow the client's arm to be easily extended. When the client's chair is too close to the manicure table, the manicurist's elbow bends sharply and the shoulder becomes raised, thereby causing undue fatigue and strain.

Your Personality Chart

No one can hope to have or maintain a successful career in manicuring unless an attractive and pleasing personality is developed.

Personality is the charm revealed in your speech, appearance, behavior and manners. What you think and how you feel are expressed by speech. How you behave in school, business or social life can either add to or take away from your personality.

Personality is your greatest asset in life. It can be cultivated by giving careful attention to details in grooming and the forming of good habits and desirable traits.

Try to make this personality chart a true picture of your inner and outer self. Study yourself first. If your rating is low, consult your teacher, friends or doctor to find out what can be done to improve it. Analyze your personality every three months to find out what progress you are making.

Personality Quiz

Check the proper box in this personality chart to find out if you have the personality qualities listed below:

Answer One

	Always	Some- times	Never
1. Do you give careful attention to personal grooming such as clothes, hair, makeup, hose and shoes?	☐	☐	☐
2. Do you sit, stand and walk with correct posture?	☐	☐	☐
3. Do you change undergarmets regularly and avoid bad breath and body odors at all times?	☐	☐	☐

4. Are you loyal to others?   □ □ □

5. Are you friendly and courteous to others?   □ □ □

6. Are you truthful in dealing with others?   □ □ □

7. Can you get along and work with others?   □ □ □

8. Can you accept responsibility?   □ □ □

9. Do you have confidence in your knowledge and
   ability?   □ □ □

10. Do you have a good tone of voice and choice of
    words?   □ □ □

To rate your personality, give yourself 10 points for *Always;* 5 points for *Sometimes;* and zero (0) for *Never.* Compare the final rating with the following standards:

Excellent Personality 85-100%

Good Personality 75-85%

Fair Personality 60-75%

Poor Personality . . . . .59% or less

HYGIENE: A Review

1. **Define the following:** a) **Hygiene.** b) **Personal Hygiene.** c) **Public Hygiene.**	a) Hygiene is the science that deals with the preservation of health. b) Personal hygiene deals with the preservation of health of the individual. c) Public hygiene deals with the promotion of public health.
2. **In what manner is the complexion an expression of health?**	b) The complexion is the outward expression of inner health.
3. **Why is cleanliness essential?**	Cleanliness is the first step towards perfect health; lack of cleanliness may be a disease-producing factor.
4. a) **Why should the skin of the body be kept clean?** b) **How should the skin of the body be kept clean?**	a) The skin should be kept clean to remove dirt and body wastes. b) The skin should be kept clean by daily bathing.
5. a) **What are the essentials of mouth hygiene?** b) **How should the teeth be taken care of?**	a) Keeping the teeth and gums in good condition and the breath sweet. b) The teeth should be brushed twice daily; they should be examined by a dentist at least twice a year, and all decayed teeth filled or removed.
6. **Why are regular physical examinations necessary?**	To keep a check on the health of the body.
7. **How may body odors be eliminated?**	By daily bathing, the use of deodorants, and regular change of garments.
8. **How is bad or offensive breath treated?**	By gargling with an antiseptic preparation. If doing so does not correct the condition, consult a dentist or physician.
9. **Why is it important that the manicurist be in good health?**	That she may be able to attend to work properly, and avoid the spreading of disease germs.
10. **What type of disease should prevent a person from working in a beauty salon?**	A person suffering from any infectious or contagious disease in any communicable form should not be allowed to work in a beauty salon.

11. When should a manicurist wash her hands?	Before and after serving each client and after each visit to the toilet.
12. What type of dress should a manicurist wear in the shop?	The manicurist should wear a clean washable uniform at all times.

PERSONALITY: A Review

1. What is personality?	Personal charm as shown by speech, behavior, appearance and manners.
2. How should the manicurist improve his or her personality?	Practice the habits of good character, vibrant health and careful grooming.
3. What is salon conduct?	The attitude and actions of the manicurist towards work, clients, co-workers, owner or manager.
4. How should the manicurist improve his or her salon conduct?	By being punctual, courteous, honest, respectful, fair and loyal. By working willingly and efficiently. By avoiding gossip.
5. What are the essentials of good grooming?	Cleanliness and neatness in regard to the skin, hair, hands, nails, makeup and fitness of your clothes.

Bacteriology, Sterilization and Sanitation

Sterilization and sanitation are subjects of practical importance to the manicurist because they have a direct bearing on the manicurist's as well as the client's welfare. To protect individual and public health, the manicurist should know when, why and how to utilize sterilization *(ster-il-i-zay'shun)* and sanitation *(san-i-tay'shun)*.

BACTERIOLOGY

Bacteriology *(bak-tir-ee-ol'o-jee)* is the science which deals with the study of micro-organisms *(my'kro-or'gan-izms)* called bacteria *(bak-tir'ee-a)*.

The manicurist must understand how the spread of disease can be prevented, and become familiar with the precautions which must be taken to protect his or her own as well as the client's health. Contagious diseases, skin infections and blood poisoning are caused either by the conveyance of infectious material from one individual to another, or by implements (such as cuticle nippers, pusher, nail file, etc.) which have been used first on an infected person and then on another, without having been sanitized.

Bacteria are minute, one-celled vegetable micro-organisms found nearly everywhere. They are especially numerous in dust, dirt, refuse and diseased tissues. Ordinarily, bacteria are not visible except with the aid of a microscope. Fifteen hundred rod-shaped bacteria will barely reach across a pinhead. It is only when thousands of them have grown in one spot to form a "colony" that they become visible as a mass.

Types of Bacteria

1. **Non-pathogenic** *(non-path-o-jen'ik)* **organisms** (beneficial type) constitute the majority of all bacteria and perform many useful functions, such as decomposing refuse and improving the fertility of the soil. To this group belong the *saprophytes* which live on dead matter.

2. **Pathogenic** *(path-o-jen'ik)* **organisms** *(microbes or germs)*, (harmful type), although in the minority, produce considerable damage by invading plant or animal tissues. Pathogenic bacteria are harmful because they produce disease. To this group belong the *parasites*, which require living matter for their growth.

It is due to pathogenic bacteria that the practice of sanitation is necessary to the manicurist.

Classification of Pathogenic Bacteria

There are hundreds of different kinds of bacteria. Pathogenic bacteria are classified into three main groups, as follows:

1. **Cocci** *(kok'see)* (singular, *coccus)* are round-shaped organisms which appear singly or in groups as follows:
   a) **Staphylococci** *(staf-i-lo-kok'see)* (singular, *staphylococcus)* are pus-forming organisms which grow in bunches or clusters, and are present in abscesses, pustules and boils.
   b) **Streptococci** *(strep-to-kok'see)* (singular, *streptococcus)* are pus-forming organisms which grow in chains, as found in blood poisoning.
   c) **Diplococci** *(dip-lo-kok'see)* (singular, *diplococcus)* grow in pairs, and cause pneumonia.
2. **Bacilli** *(bah-sil'i)* (singular, *bacillus)* are rod-shaped organisms. They are the most common and produce such diseases as tetanus (lockjaw), influenza, typhoid, tuberculosis and diphtheria. Many bacilli are *spore* producers.
3. **Spiralla** *(spi-ril'ah)* (singular, *spirillum)* are curved or corkscrew-shaped organisms. They are further subdivided into several groups, of chief importance being the *spirochaetal* organisms. The *spirochaeta* called *Treponema pallida* is the causative agent in *syphilis.*

Bacterial Growth and Reproduction

Germs live, grow and multiply best in warm, dark damp and dirty places where sufficient food is present. Many parts of the human body offer a suitable breeding place for bacteria.

THREE GENERAL FORMS OF BACTERIA

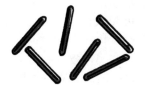
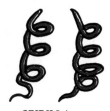

COCCI	*BACILLI*	*SPIRILLA*

GROUPINGS OF BACTERIA

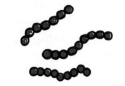

DIPLOCOCCI	*STREPTOCOCCI*	*STAPHYLOCOCCI*

SIX DISEASE-PRODUCING BACTERIA

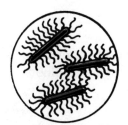
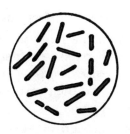
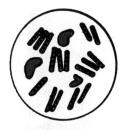

TYPHOID BACILLUS
SHOWING FLAGELLA

TUBERCLE BACILLUS
(Tuberculosis)

DIPHTHERIA
BACILLUS

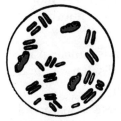
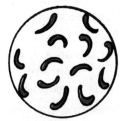
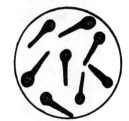

INFLUENZA
BACILLUS

CHOLERA
(Microspira)

TETANUS BACILLUS
WITH SPORES

TO AVOID THE SPREAD OF DISEASE
Keep yourself clean. Keep your surroundings clean. Keep everything you come in contact with clean. Make sure that everything you use is clean.

When conditions are favorable, bacteria reproduce very fast. As food is absorbed, the bacterium cell grows in size. When the limit of growth is reached, it divides crosswise into halves, thereby forming two daughter cells. From one bacterium, as many as 16 million germs may develop in half a day.

Spore-forming bacteria. When favorable conditions cease to exist, bacteria either die or cease to multiply. To withstand periods of famine, dryness and unsuitable temperature, certain bacteria such as the anthrax and tetanus bacilli can form spherical spores having a tough outer covering. In this stage, the spore can be blown about in the dust and is not harmed by disinfectants, heat or cold.

When favorable conditions are restored, the spore becomes active again and starts to grow and reproduce.

Movement of Bacteria

The ability to move about is limited to the bacilli and spiralla, which have hair-like projections, known as *flagella (fla-jel'a)* or *cilia (sil'ee-a)*. By moving these fine hairs with a whip-like motion, these bacteria propel themselves about through a liquid.

Bacterial Infections

An *infection* occurs when the body is unable to cope with the bacteria and their harmful toxins. At first, the infection may be *localized*, as in a boil. A *general infection* results when the bloodstream carries the bacteria and their toxins to all parts of the body, as in blood poisoning or syphilis.

The presence of pus is a sign of infection. Found in pus are bacteria, body cells and blood cells, both living and dead.

An infectious disease becomes *contagious (kon-tay'jus)* when it tends to spread more or less readily from one person to another by direct or indirect contact.

The chief sources of contagion are: unclean hands, unclean instruments, open sores and pus, mouth and nose discharges, and the common use of drinking cups and towels.

Uncovered coughing, sneezing and spitting in public also spread germs. Through personal hygiene and public sanitation, infections can be prevented and controlled.

The body fights infections with its defensive forces. The first line of defense is the unbroken skin. In a healthy person, body secretions such as perspiration and digestive juices discourage bacterial growth. Within the blood, there are white corpuscles to devour bacteria, and antitoxins to counteract the toxins produced by the bacteria.

Other Infectious Agents

Filterable viruses *(fil'ter-a-bl vy'ru-sez)* are living organisms so small that they will pass through the pores of a porcelain filter. They cause polio, influenza, smallpox, rabies, and the comon cold.

Rickettsia are much smaller than ordinary germs but are larger than viruses. They cause diseases, such as typhus and Rocky Mountain spotted fever. Fleas, ticks and lice can transmit and infect man with rickettsia.

Fungi *(fun'jy)* are microscopic plant organisms consisting of many cells, such as molds, mildews and yeast. Fungi are incapable of manufacturing their own food and behave either as parasites *(par'a-sites)* or saprophytes *(sap'ro-fites)*. Ringworm and favus are typical diseases caused by parasitic fungi.

Protozoa *(pro-to-zo'a)* are one-celled animal organisms characterized by their distinct nuclei. There are various kinds of protozoa, among which are the parasites.

Animal parasites, consisting of many cells and belonging to the insect class, are responsible for such contagious diseases as scabies due to the itch-mite, and pediculosis caused by lice.

Bacteria and other infectious agents can enter the body through any of the following routes:
1. Through the mouth (with food, water and air).
2. Through the nose (with air).
3. Through the eyes (on dirt).
4. Through breaks or wounds in the skin.

Immunity

Immunity is the ability of the body to resist disease and destroy bacteria once they have gained entrance. Immunity against disease is a sign of good health. It may be natural or acquired. *Natural immunity* is partly inherited and partly developed by hygienic living. *Acquired immunity* is secured after the body has by itself overcome certain diseases, or when it has been assisted by injection of a serum or vaccine.

Human Disease Carrier

A person may be immune to a disease and yet harbor germs which can infect other people. Such a person is called a *human disease carrier*. The diseases most frequently transmitted in this manner are typhoid fever and diphtheria.

Destruction of Bacteria

The destruction of bacteria may be accomplished by the use of disinfectants, intense heat (such as boiling water, steaming, baking or burning), or exposure to ultraviolet rays.

BACTERIOLOGY: A Review

1. Define bacteriology	Bacteriology is the science or study of bacteria.
2. What are bacteria?	Bacteria are minute, one-celled vegetable micro-organisms found nearly everywhere.
3. Name and briefly describe two types of bacteria.	Non-pathogenic bacteria—non-disease-producing, beneficial or harmless type. Pathogenic bacteria—disease-producing, and harmful type.
4. Why are bacteria not visible to the naked eye?	Because they are so minute; 15 hundred rod-shaped bacteria barely reach across a pin-head.
5. Name three general forms of bacteria, and the shape of each.	Coccus—round shape. Bacillus—rod shape. Spirillum—corkscrew shape.
6. Name four principal routes through which bacteria may enter the body.	Through the mouth, nose, eyes and through breaks or wounds in the skin.
7. How do bacteria multiply?	Bacteria multiply by each organism lengthening itself and dividing in the middle, forming two daughter cells which grow to full size and then reproduce.
8. Name two common pus-forming bacteria.	Staphylococcus and streptococcus.
9. Why does the manicurist study bacteria in connection with sanitation?	Because pathogenic bacteria are harmful and disease producers, the knowledge of sanitation is necessary.

10. **Define the following terms:**
    a) pathogenic.
    b) non-pathogenic.

a) Pathogenic means disease-producing.
b) Non-pathogenic means non-disease-producing, beneficial or harmless.

11. **a) What is a communicable disease?**
    b) Name two.

a) A communicable disease is one that may be transmitted from one person to another.
b) Influenza and common cold.

12. **What will destroy bacteria?**

Disinfectants, intense heat, such as boiling, steaming, baking or burning, or exposure to ultraviolet rays.

13. **What is the difference between natural and acquired immunity?**

Natural immunity means natural resistance to disease. Acquired immunity is secured after the body has by itself overcome certain diseases, or has been assisted by injection of serum or vaccine.

STERILIZATION AND SANITATION

Sterilization is the process of making an object germ-free by the destruction of all kinds of bacteria, whether beneficial or harmful.

Sterilization and sanitation are of practical importance to the manicurist because they deal with methods used to prevent the growth of germs or destroy them entirely, particularly those which are responsible for infections and communicable diseases.

Health departments and state boards of cosmetology recognize that it is impossible to completely sterilize all implements and equipment in the beauty salon. Therefore, it is generally recognized that implements and equipment are *sanitized* and not sterilized.

Throughout the entire text the term "sanitize" will be used to indicate all forms of sanitation.

The manicurist should obey the rules on sanitation issued by the health department and state board of cosmetology regarding acceptable methods of sanitation.

Methods of Sanitation

There are many methods of sanitation with which the manicurist should be familiar. These may be grouped under two main headings:

1. Physical agents:
   Ultraviolet rays.

2. Chemical agents:
   a) Antiseptics and disinfectants.
   b) Vapors (fumigation).

Physical Agents

Ultraviolet rays. Bacteria cannot tolerate the effect of direct sunlight for more than a few hours. Almost all bacteria may be killed or weakened by **ultraviolet irradiation.**

Chemical Agents

Chemicals are the most effective sanitizing agents that may be used in beauty salons in destroying or slowing the growth of bacteria. The chemical agents used for sanitizing purposes are either antiseptics *(an'ti-sep'tiks)* or disinfectants *(dis-in-fek'tants)* (germicides) *(jer'mi-sides)*. A distinction is usually made between an antiseptic and a disinfectant.

1. An **antiseptic** is a substance which may kill or retard the growth of bacteria without killing them. Antiseptics can be used with safety on the skin.

2. A **disinfectant** destroys bacteria and is used for the sanitization of instruments.

Chemicals such as alcohol or "quats" can be classed under both heads: a *strong solution* may be used as a disinfectant and a *weak solution* as an antiseptic.

Wet Sanitizer

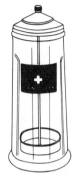

A wet sanitizer is any receptacle large enough to hold the disinfectant solution and completely immerse the objects to be sanitized. A cover is provided to prevent contamination of the solution. Wet sanitizers come in various sizes and shapes.

Before immersing objects in a wet sanitizer containing a disinfectant solution, throughly cleanse them with soap and water. This procedure removes most of the bacteria and prevents contamination of the solution.

Wet sanitizer.

After the implements are removed from the disinfectant solution, they should be rinsed in clean water, wiped dry with a clean towel and stored in a dry or cabinet sanitizer until ready to be used.

Dry (Cabinet) Sanitizer

Dry or cabinet sanitizer is an air-tight cabinet containing an active fumigant (formaldehyde gas). The sterilized implements are kept sanitary by placing them in the cabinet until ready for use.

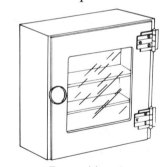

How the fumigant *(fyu'mi-gant)* **is prepared.** Place one tablespoonful of borax and one tablespoonful of formalin on a small tray or blotter on the bottom of the cabinet. This will form formaldehyde vapors. Replace chemicals regularly; they lose their strength after a few days. Formaldehyde tablets are also available now.

Dry sanitizer.

Ultraviolet ray electrical sanitizers are effective for keeping implements clean until ready for use. Implements must be sanitized before they are placed in the ultraviolet sanitizer. Follow manufacturer's directions for proper use.

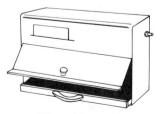

Ultra-violet sanitizer.

PROPORTIONS FOR MAKING PERCENTAGE SOLUTIONS

100% Active Liquid Concentrate   **Strength**
5 drops of liquid to 1 oz (30 ml) water or
1 teaspoon (5 ml) of liquid to 12 oz. (.36 l) water 1%
10 drops of liquid to 1 oz. (30 ml) water or
2 teaspoonfuls (10 ml) of liquid to 12 oz. (.36 l) water 2%
4 teaspoonfuls (20 ml) of liquid to 12 oz. (.36 l) water 4%
5 teaspoonfuls (25 ml) of liquid to 12 oz. (.36 l) water 5%
10 teaspoonfuls (50 ml) of liquid to 12 oz. (.36 l) water 10%

Table of Equivalents
Ordinary measured glass . . . . 8 oz. (.237 l)
1 pint. . . . . .16 oz. (.475 l)
1 quart . . . . .32 oz. (.95 l)
½ gallon . . . . .64 oz. (1.9l)

CHEMICAL SANITIZING AGENTS
Quaternary Ammonium Compounds ("Quats")

Quaternary ammonium compounds *(kwa-ter'na-ree a-mone'ee-um kom'powndz)* are a broad range of surface-active chemical agents of importance in the salon. "Quats" *(kwats)* are formulated into products that you will be using as disinfectants, cleansers, sterilizers, and fungicides for sanitation purposes that we will discuss in this chapter. Quats can also be formulated into cleansers, hand lotions, and various conditioning products that we will discuss in later chapters.

The advantages claimed for quats as a sanitation agent are that they offer a short disinfection time and are odorless, colorless, non-toxic, and stable. A 1:1000 solution is commonly used to sanitize implements. Immersion time ranges from 1-5 minutes, depending on the strength of the solution used.

How to Prepare a 1:1000 Strength Solution of a Quaternary Ammonium Compound
If the product contains:
10% active ingredient, add 1¼ oz (37.5 ml) quat solution to 1 gallon (3.8 l) of water.

12½% active ingredient, add 1 oz. (30 ml) quat solution to 1 gallon (3.8 l) of water.

15% active ingredient, add ¾ oz. (22.5 ml) quat solution to 1 gallon (3.8 l) of water.

Sanitation with Quats and Other Chemical Disinfectants

1. Wash implements thoroughly with soap and warm water.
2. Use final plain water rinse to remove all traces of soap.
3. Immerse implements into wet sanitizer (containing quats or other approved disinfectant) for the required time.*
4. Remove implements from wet sanitizer, rinse in water and wipe dry with clean towel.
5. Store sanitized implements in individually wrapped cellophane envelopes or keep in cabinet sanitizer until ready to be used.

Sanitation with Formalin

Formalin is an effective sanitizing agent which can be used as a disinfectant. As purchased, formalin is approximately 37% to 40% of formaldehyde gas in water. Formalin should be used with great care, because inhalation can cause damage to mucous membranes, and contact with the skin can cause irritation. Due to its potential harm, formalin is most commonly added to prepared sanitizing agents and used in various strengths, as follows:

25% solution (equivalent to 10% formaldehyde) is used to sanitize instruments. Immerse them in the solution for at least 10 minutes. (Preparation: 2 parts formalin, 5 parts water, 1 part glycerine.)

10% solution (equivalent to 4% formaldehyde) is used to sanitize combs and brushes. Immerse them for at least 20 minutes. (Preparation: 1 part formalin, 9 parts water.)

Sanitation with Alcohol

To sanitize **manicuring** or other **implements,** immerse them in 70% alcohol for 10 or more minutes.

Instruments having a fine cutting edge are best sanitized by rubbing the surface with a cotton pad dampened in 70% alcohol, which prevents the cutting edges from becoming dull.

Electrodes may be safely sanitized by gently rubbing the exposed surface with a cotton pad dampened in 70% alcohol.

Sanitation with Sodium Hypochlorite

With the advent of the AIDS virus comes the addition of the sodium hypochlorite compounds (household bleach). These are

---

*Consult your state board of cosmetology or health department for list of approved disinfectants to be used in beauty salons.

agents that have been included in many commercially available sanitizing agents. The pure compound, common household bleach, can be used in the school or salon. Manicuring implements should be immersed in a 10% solution of sodium hypochlorite for 10 or more minutes.

Sanitizing Floors, Sinks and Toilet Bowls
The disinfection of floors, sinks and toilet bowls in the beauty salon calls for the use of commercial products such as Lysol, pine needle oil or similar disinfectants. Deodorants are also useful to off-set offensive odors and for imparting a refreshing odor. Whatever disinfectant is being used, make sure that it is properly diluted as suggested by the manufacturer.

What Is An Approved Disinfectant?
Consult with your state board of cosmetology or health department for a list of approved disinfectants to be used in the school. You will find the following chemicals:

NAME	FORM	STRENGTH	HOW TO USE
Sodium Hypochlorite (household bleach)	Liquid	10% solution	Immerse implements in solution for 10 or more minutes.
Quaternary Ammonium Compounds	Liquid or tablet	1:1000 solution	Immerse implements in solution for 20 or more minutes.
Formalin	Liquid	25% solution	Immerse implements in solution for 10 or more minutes.
Formalin	Liquid	10% solution	Immerse implements in solution for 20 or more minutes.
Alcohol	Liquid	70% solution	Immerse implements or sanitize electrodes and sharp cutting edges 10 or more minutes.

Safety Precautions
The use of chemical agents for sanitation involves certain dangers, unless safety measures are taken to prevent mistakes and accidents.

1. Purchase chemicals in small quantities and store them in a cool, dry place; otherwise, they deteriorate upon contact with air, light and heat.

2. Weigh and measure chemicals carefully.

3. Keep all containers labeled and covered under lock and key.

4. Do not smell chemicals or solutions, as many of them have pungent odors and can cause lung damage.

5. Avoid spilling when dissolving or diluting chemicals.

6. Keep a complete first aid kit on hand.

Definitions Pertaining to Sanitation

1. **Sterilize**—to render sterile; to make free from all bacteria (harmful or beneficial).

2. **Sterile**—free from all living organisms.

3. **Antiseptic**—a chemical agent having the power to kill or retard the growth of bacteria.

4. **Germicide** *(Bactericide* or *Disinfectant)*—a chemical agent having the power to destroy germs or microbes.

5. **Deodorant**—a chemical agent having the power to destroy offensive odors.

6. **Asepsis** *(aye-sep'sis)*—freedom from disease germs.

7. **Sepsis**—poisoning due to pathogenic bacteria.

8. **Styptic**—an agent causing contraction of living tissue, such as powdered alum; used to stop bleeding in cases of small cuts.

9. **Fumigant**—a vapor used to keep disinfected objects sterile.

10. **Sanitize**—to render clean or sanitary.

Public Regulations and Rules of Sanitation

Sanitation is the application of measures to promote public health and prevent the spread of infectious diseases. Every manicurist should be familiar with the state's sanitation regulations governing manicuring. A manicurist with a contagious illness or disease should not serve a client. Likewise, a client suffering from such illnesses should not be handled by the manicurist.

Sanitation Rules in Manicuring

The manicurist has the responsibility of sanitizing all manicure instruments prior to using them on the client. Following their use, these tools are to be sanitized and kept ready for the next manicure.

To save time, two sets of tools should be available. While one set is in use, the other set remains sanitized in the cabinet sanitizer.

To protect the client's welfare, the manicurist should obey the following rules of sanitation:

1. Wear a clean uniform at all times.

2. Wash hands throughly before an after each manicure and after leaving the toilet.

3. Use a clean, sanitized towel for each client.

4. Sanitize manicure instruments after each use.
   a) Wash instruments in hot soapy water. Files and nippers should be wiped with alcohol to clear them of particles of nail or skin.
   b) Rinse and immerse them in sanitizing solution.
   c) Rinse, dry and place instruments in dry sanitizer until used.

5. To prevent deterioration, change chemical solution in sanitizers regularly.

6. The use of the same styptic pencil by more than one person is prohibited. Provide individual paper cups for finger bowls.

7. Lotions, ointments and creams must be kept in clean, closed containers.

8. Use sanitized spatula to remove cosmetics from jars. Use clean cotton pledgets to apply lotions and powders.

9. Objects dropped on the floor are not to be used until sanitized.

10. Before use, all linens, instruments and articles must be sanitized and then placed in a dust-proof or air tight container or a cabinet sanitizer.

STERILIZATION AND SANITATION: A Review

Note: The immersion of implements in a chemical solution should conform to state board of cosmetology regulations issued by your state.

Sterilization and Sanitation

1. What is sterilization?	Sterilization is the process of completely destroying all kinds of bacteria, whether harmful or beneficial.
2. Name the methods of sanitation.	Physical agents, such as ultraviolet rays, and chemical agents, such as disinfectants, antiseptics and vapors.

3. **Which type of bacteria makes necessary the practice of sanitation in the beauty salon?**

Pathogenic bacteria.

4. **What are the dangers of using unsanitized implements and linens on clients?**

Infectious diseases may be spread from one person to another.

5. **Distinguish between asepsis, sterile and sepsis.**

Asepsis—freedom from germs.
Sterile—free from all living organisms.
Sepsis—poisoning due to germs.

6. **Which groups of chemicals will slow the growth of or destroy bacteria?**

Antiseptics, disinfectants, and fumigants.

7. **What is an antiseptic?**

A chemical agent which may kill or prevent the growth of bacteria.

8. **What is a disinfectant?**

A chemical agent which destroys harmful bacteria.

9. **What is a fumigant in a dry sanitizer?**

A chemical vapor used to keep disinfected objects in a sanitary condition until ready for use.

10. **What are four advantages of using "quats" as a disinfectant?**

Quats have a short disinfection time and are odorless, nontoxic and stable.

11. **In measuring liquids:**
   a) How many teaspoonfuls equal 1 oz?
   b) How many ounces equal 1 pint?

a) 8 teaspoonfuls.
b) 16 ozs.

12. **What is a wet sanitizer, and how is it best used?**

A wet sanitizer, is a receptacle containing a disinfectant solution. Immerse clean implements into wet sanitizer for required time.

13. **When using a disinfectant, how are objects sanitized?**

Clean each object with soap and hot water and place it into a suitable disinfectant solution for required time.

14. **What should be done with implements after sanitation in a disinfectant solution?**

Rinse implements in clean water, dry them in a clean towel and place them in a cabinet sanitizer until ready to be used.

15. **What is a dry sanitizer?**

A closed air-tight cabinet containing an active fumigant (formaldehyde gas).

16. **What is the proper way to produce formaldehyde vapors in a cabinet sanitizer?**	Place one tablespoon of borax and one tablespoon of formalin solution on a small tray or blotter on the bottom of cabinet sanitizer.
17. **What is the composition of formalin?**	Formalin is a 37% to 40% solution of formaldehyde gas dissolved in water.
18. **What is the best way to sanitize sharp implements and prevent their dulling?**	Rub the surface and sharp edges with a cotton pad dampened in 70% alcohol.
19. **What strengths of the following sanitizers are used?** **a) Alcohol** **b) Formalin** **c) "Quats"**	a) 70% alcohol b) 10%-25% formalin c) 1:1000 solution

Regulations and Rules of Sanitation

1. **Define sanitation.**	Sanitation refers to the employment of measures designed to promote public health and prevent disease.
2. **Why should there be public control over sanitary conditions in beauty salons?**	To control or prevent the spread of disease due to unsanitary conditions.
3. **Which do you consider the two most important of the sanitary rules and regulations?**	The sanitizing of all implements and articles, and washing of the hands before and after serving each client.
4. **How often should the manicurist cleanse his or her hands?**	Before and after giving a manicure, and after leaving the toilet.
5. **What is the objection to the use of the common towel?**	It is one of the most common means of transmitting disease.
6. **Name a list of articles found in a beauty salon that help to keep it sanitary.**	Wet and dry sanitizers, disinfectant and antiseptic solutions, towel cabinet, and hot and cold running water.
7. **What is the sanitary regulations governing the sanitizing of all towels used in a beauty salon?**	All towels must be laundered after use on each client and then placed in an air-tight, dust-proof cabinet until used again.

The Nail

The condition of the **nail,** like that of the skin, reflects the general health of the body. The normal, healthy nail is firm and flexible and appears to be slightly pink in color. Its surface is smooth, curved, and unspotted, without any hollows or wavy ridges.

The **nail,** an appendage of the skin, is a horny, translucent plate that protects the tips of the fingers and toes. **Onyx** *(on'iks)* is the technical term for nail.

Composition. The nail is composed mainly of **keratin** *(ker'ah-tin),* a protein substance that forms the base of all horny tissue. The nail is whitish in appearance and allows the pinkish color of the nail bed to be seen. The horny nail plate contains no nerves or blood vessels.

Nail Structure

The nails consist of three parts: nail body, nail root, and free edge.

The **nail body,** or **plate,** is the visible portion of the nail that rests upon, and is attached to, the **nail bed.** The nail body extends from the **root** to the **free edge.**

Although the nail plate seems to be one piece, it is actually constructed in layers. The readiness with which nails split, in both their length and thickness, clearly shows this form of structure.

The **nail root** is at the base of the nail and is embedded underneath the skin. It originates from an actively growing tissue known as the **matrix** *(may'triks).*

The **free edge** is the end portion of the nail plate that reaches over the fingertip.

Structures Adjoining The Nail

Nail Bed

The **nail bed** is the portion of the skin upon which the nail body rests. It is supplied with many blood vessels which provide the nourishment necessary for the continued growth of the nail. The nail bed is abundantly supplied with nerves.

Matrix

The **matrix** is that part of the nail bed that extends beneath the nail root and contains nerves, lymph, and blood vessels. The matrix produces the nail as its cells undergo a reproducing and hardening process. The matrix will continue to grow as long as it receives nutrition and remains in a healthy condition.

However, the growth of the nails may be retarded if an individual is in poor health, if a nail disorder or disease is present, or if there is an injury to the nail matrix.

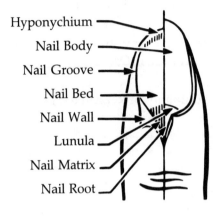

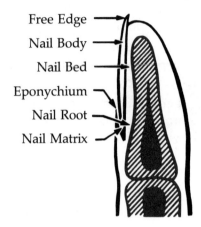

DIAGRAM OF A NAIL   CROSS-SECTION OF A NAIL

Lunula

The **lunula** *(loo'nyu-la)*, or *half-moon*, is located at the base of the nail. The area underneath the lunula is the matrix. The light color of the lunula may be due to the reflection of light where the matrix and the connective tissue of the nail bed join.

Parts Surrounding The Nail

The **cuticle** (kyu'ti-kl) is the overlapping epidermis around the nail. A normal cuticle should be loose and pliable.

The **eponychium** *(ep-o-nik'ee-um)* is the extension of the cuticle at the base of the nail body which partly overlaps the lunula.

The **hyponychium** *(hy-po-nik'ee-um)* is that portion of the epidermis under the free edge of the nail.

The **perionychium** *(per-i-o-nik'ee-um)* is that portion of the cuticle surrounding the entire nail border.

The **nail walls** are the folds of skin overlapping the sides of the nail.

The **nail grooves** are slits, or tracks, on the sides of the nail upon which the nail moves as it grows.

The **mantle** *(man'tl)* is the deep fold of skin in which the nail root is embedded.

Nail Growth

The growth of the nail is influenced by nutrition, health, and disease. The nail grows forward, starting at the matrix and extending over the tip of the finger.

The average rate of growth in the normal adult is about 1/8" (.3125 cm) per month, growing faster in the summer than in the winter. The nails of children grow more rapidly, whereas those of elderly persons grow more slowly. The nail grows fastest on the middle finger and slowest on the thumb. Toenails grow more slowly than fingernails, and are thicker and harder.

Nail Malformation

If the nail is separated from the nail bed through injury, it becomes distorted or discolored. Should the nail bed be injured after the loss of a nail, a badly formed nail will result.

The nails are neither shed automatically nor periodically, as are hairs. If the nail is torn off accidentally, or lost through an infection or disease, it will be replaced only as long as the matrix remains in good condition. Nails lost under such conditions are, on regrowth, frequently badly shaped, due to interference at the base of the nail. Ordinarily, replacement of the nail takes about four months.

Various Shapes of Nails

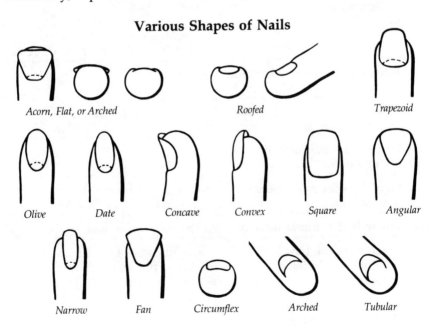

Acorn, Flat, or Arched   *Roofed*   *Trapezoid*

Olive   *Date*   *Concave*   *Convex*   *Square*   *Angular*

Narrow   *Fan*   *Circumflex*   *Arched*   *Tubular*

THE NAIL: A Review

1. Describe the appearance of a healthy nail.	A healthy nail is firm and flexible and appears to be slightly pink in color. Its surface is smooth, curved, and unspotted, without any hollows or wavy ridges.
2. What are nails?	Nails are horny, translucent plates.
3. What is the main function of the nail?	To protect the tips of the fingers and toes.
4. What is the technical term for nail?	Onyx.
5. Of what is the nail composed?	A nail is composed mainly of keratin, a protein substance.
6. Describe the structure of the nail plate.	The nail plate seems to be one piece, but actually it is constructed in layers.
7. Locate the following: **a) nail root** **b) nail body** **c) free edge** **d) nail bed**	a) At the base of the nail, underneath the skin. b) It rests upon, and is attached to, the nail bed. c) The end portion of the nail reaching over the fingertip. d) Skin upon which nail body rests.
8. What part of the nail contains the nerve and blood supply?	The matrix.
9. What three factors retard the growth of the nail?	Poor health, nail disorder or disease, injury to the nail matrix.
10. Where does the formation of the nail occur?	In the matrix.
11. How does the nail receive its nourishment?	From the matrix, which contains nerves, lymph, and blood vessels.
12. Where is the lunula located?	At the base of the nail.
13. What gives the lunula the half-moon, whitish appearance?	The light color of the lunula may be due to the reflection of light where the matrix and the connective tissue of the nail bed join.
14. Where is the eponychium found?	Eponychium is the extension of the cuticle at the base of the nail body that partly overlaps the lunula.

15. Define the following:
   a) cuticle
   b) mantle
   c) nail grooves
	a) Cuticle is the overlapping epidermis around the nail.
	b) Mantle is the deep fold of skin in which the nail root is embedded.
	c) Nail grooves are slits on the sides of the nail upon which the nail moves as it grows.

16. What is the hyponychium?	The portion of the epidermis under the free edge.
17. Define perionychium.	The portion of the cuticle surrounding the entire nail border.
18. What two factors promote the growth of the nail?	Nutrition and health.
19. Where does nail growth start, and in which direction does it continue?	The nail grows forward, starting at the matrix and extending over the tip of the finger.
20. What is the average growth of the nail in the normal adult?	1/8″ per month.
21. If a healthy nail is torn off, will it be replaced?	Yes, if the matrix remains in good condition.

The Practice of Manicuring

Why Study the Science and Art of Manicuring?

Your success depends to a large extent on knowing the "what," the "why" and the "how" of manicuring services offered to clients.

The science of manicuring is of value to the manicurist in the following ways:

1. To provide the proper nail care to clients, the manicurist should know the nail structure and how the nail grows, and be able to detect common nail disorders.

2. To select the right product, the manicurist should now what each product is capable of doing for the client's nails, and skin of the arms and hands.

3. To give the right kind of hand and arm massage, the manicurist needs to know the structure of the arms and hands, various massage movements and their effect on the blood circulation.

Knowing the science and art of manicuring helps to build confidence. A knowledgeable, confident manicurist will attract clients who will come back again and again.

Manicuring

The ancients regarded long, polished and colored fingernails as a mark distinguishing the aristocrat from the common laborer. Manicuring, once considered a luxury for the few, is now within reach of the general public. In fact, every well-groomed person seeks regular manicures.

Manicuring is not limited to the hands of women. More and more men request the services of a manicurist when they visit the barber or styling shop or full service salon.

The word *manicuring* is derived from the Latin words *manus* (hand) and *cura* (care), meaning the care of the hands and nails. The purpose of a manicure is to improve the appearance of the hands and nails.

The cosmetologist frequently begins his or her career with manicuring. A cosmetologist's nails should exemplify a well-groomed, beautiful appearance. If the client is pleased by a good manicure, she or he is more likely to become a regular customer for manicuring as well as other salon treatments.

A qualified manicurist should have the following:
1. Knowledge of the structure of hands, arms and nails.
2. Knowledge of the composition of various cosmetics used in manicuring.
3. Ability to give a good manicure in a systematic and efficient manner.
4. Ability to care for the client's manicuring problems.
5. Ability to please and satisfy clients.
6. Ability to distinguish between disorders that may be treated in the salon and diseases that must be treated by a physician.

Equipment, Implements, Cosmetics and Materials
The articles used in manicuring, that are more or less durable or permanent, are referred to as equipment and implements or tools. Materials refer to cosmetics and other supplies that are consumed and therefore, must be replaced from time to time.

MANICURING IMPLEMENTS

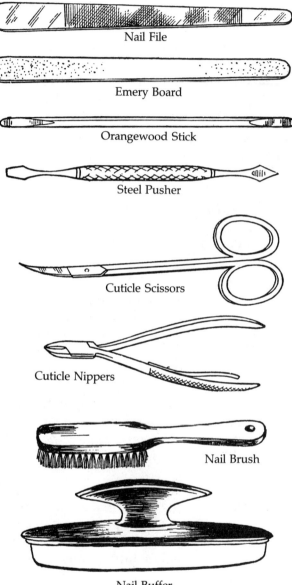

Nail File

Emery Board

Orangewood Stick

Steel Pusher

Cuticle Scissors

Cuticle Nippers

Nail Brush

Nail Buffer

Equipment

The equipment needed in giving a manicure includes:

1. **Manicure table** and adjustable lamp.

2. **Client's chair** and **manicurist's chair** or **stool.**

3. **Cushion** (8 by 12 inches) covered with washable slip or sanitized towel on which client rests arm. A Turkish towel, folded and covered with a small sanitized towel, may be used instead of the cushion.

4. **Supply tray** for holding cosmetics.

5. **Finger bowl** (plastic, china or glass, with removable paper cups) for holding warm water and cleanser.

6. **Cotton container** for absorbent sterile cotton.

7. **Electric heater** for heating oil when giving a hot oil manicure.

8. **Wet sanitizer container.**

9. **Glass containers** for cosmetics and accessories.

10. **70% alcohol**—for sanitizing implements.

Implements

Implements include the following:

1. **Orangewood sticks** (2)—to loosen cuticle and work around nail and for applying oil, cream, bleach or solvent to the nail and cuticle.

2. **Nail file** (7 or 8 inches long, thin and flexible)—to shape and smooth the free edge of the nail.

3. **Cuticle pusher**—to push back and loosen the cuticle.

4. **Cuticle nippers**—to trim the cuticle. Cuticle scissors are very seldom used professionally.

5. **Nail brush**—to cleanse the nails and fingertips with the aid of warm soapy water.

6. **Emery boards** (several)—to shape the free edge of the nail with the coarse side and to bevel the nail with the finer side.

7. **Nail buffer** (with removable frame to permit replacement of the chamois cover)—to buff and polish the nails. (Some states do not permit the use of a nail buffer.)

8. **Fine camel's-hair brush**—to apply lacquer or liquid nail polish. (Camel's-hair brush is usually attached to top of nail polish bottle.)

9. **Tweezers**—for lifting small bits of cuticle.

Cosmetics

Nail and hand cosmetics vary in their composition and usage according to the purpose they serve.

Nail cleansers consist of some form of detergent, usually liquid, flakes or a cake.

Nail polish removers contain organic solvents and are used to dissolve the old polish present on the nails. To offset the drying action of the solvent, oil may be present in the nail polish remover.

Cuticle oil softens and lubricates the skin around the nails.

Cuticle creams are usually lanolin, petroleum or beeswax based. They are intended to prevent or correct brittle nails and dry cuticle.

Cuticle removers or solvents may contain sodium or potassium hydroxide plus glycerine. Milder solutions may instead contain trisodium and triethanolamine or alkanolamines. After the cuticle is softened with this liquid, it can be easily removed.

Nail bleachers contain hydrogen peroxide or dilute organic acids in a liquid form or mixed with other ingredients to form a white paste. When applied over nails, under the free edge of the nail and on fingertips, stains are removed.

Abrasives are available as a pumice powder or stone, and are used to smooth irregular nail ridges.

Nail whiteners are applied as a paste, cream, coated string or special white pencil. They consists mainly of white pigments (zinc oxide or titanium dioxide). When applied under the nails, they keep the tips looking white.

Dry nail polish is usually prepared in the form of powder or paste. The main ingredient is a mild abrasive, such as tin oxide or pumice powder. It smooths the nail and also imparts a sheen to the nail during buffing.

Liquid nail polish or lacquer is used to color or gloss the nail. It is a solution of nitro cellulose in such volatile solvents as **amyl acetate,** together with a **plasticiser** (castor oil), which prevent too rapid drying.

Nail polish solvent is used to thin out the nail polish.

A base coat is a liquid product applied before the liquid nail polish. With this application, the nail polish adheres readily to the nail surface.

A **top coat** or sealer is a liquid product applied over the nail polish. It imparts toughness and extra gloss, and makes the nail polish more resistant to chipping.

A **nail dryer** is a fine spray which protects the nail polish against tackiness and dulling. Can be used either as a spray over the top coat or directly on the nail polish.

Hand creams and lotions keep the skin soft by replacing the natural oils lost from the skin. They are recommended for overcoming a dry, chapped or irritated condition of the skin.

Hand creams are made up of emollients, humectants (such as glycerine or propylene glycol), which promote the retention of water, emulsifiers and preservatives.

Hand lotions are similar in composition to hand creams, but they possess a thinner consistency due to a higher oil content.

Materials

Materials include the following articles:

1. **Absorbent cotton**—to apply cosmetics to the nails.
2. **Cleanser** (liquid or any form)—for finger bath.
3. **Warm water**—for finger bath.
4. **Sanitized towels**—use individual towel for each client.
5. **Cleansing tissue**—to use whenever necessary.
6. **Chamois**—to replace soiled chamois on buffer.
7. **Paper cups**—to replace used paper cups in finger bowl.
8. **Antiseptic**—to add a few drops to bath; to apply on minor injuries to tissues surrounding the nails.
9. **Disinfectant**—to sanitize instruments; to sponge the manicure table.
10. **Spatula**—to remove creams from jars.
11. **Mending tissue paper**—to repair or cover broken, split or torn nails.
12. **70% alcohol**—to sanitize implements during a manicure, or to sanitize client's fingers before a manicure.
13. **Powdered alum or alum solution**—to stop the bleeding of minor cuts.

Preparation of the Manicuring Table

To give a professional manicure, all rules of sanitation must be followed. The table and the manicurist's hands must be perfectly clean. Everything, including containers, bowls, instruments, and materials, must be in perfect order. Do not ask the client to sit at the table with the remains of the previous manicure in sight. Always clean the table immediately upon completion of a manicure so that it will be ready for the next client. This will make the manicure more pleasing to the client, and will put him or her in a more receptive mood for your advice and suggestions.

Procedure

1. Sponge the manicuring tabletop with a disinfectant.
2. Place a clean towel over the armrest or cushion.
3. Place a bowl of warm, soapy water to the left of the client.
4. Place the metal implements and orangewood sticks in a jar sanitizer containing cotton saturated with alcohol.
5. Arrange cream jars, lotion bottles, and nail polishes in the order to be used and place them to the left of the manicurist.
6. Place the nail file (which has been sponged with alcohol) and fresh emery boards to the right of the manicurist.
7. Attach a small plastic bag to the table with Scotch tape, on either the right or left side, for waste materials.

Manicuring Table Setup

(Your instructor's manicuring table setup is equally correct.)

1. *Towel wrapped armrest*
2. *Nail file*
3. *Emery board*
4. *Alcohol*
5. *Cotton container*
6. *Finger bowl*
7. *Nail brush*
8. *Wet sanitizer containing manicuring implements*
9. *Tray with nail polishes*

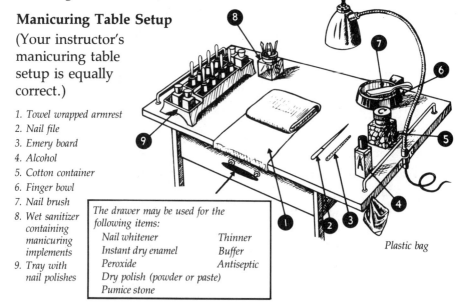

The drawer may be used for the following items:

Nail whitener	*Thinner*
Instant dry enamel	*Buffer*
Peroxide	*Antiseptic*
Dry polish (powder or paste)	
Pumice stone	

Plastic bag

The manicuring table drawer always should be clean and neat. Do not use it for waste materials; use the plastic bag.

Shapes of Nails

Nails naturally vary greatly in shape, but are usually classified into four general shapes: **square, oval, pointed** and **round.** In selecting the nail shape best suited for the client, consult her wishes and give consideration to the type of finger the client has. For a short, stumpy finger, a long, oval-shaped nail is to be recommended. A long, tapering finger requires a short, slightly curved nail.

The shape of the nail should conform to that of the fingertips for a more natural effect. In general, the oval-shaped nail, nicely rounded at the base, and slightly pointed at the tips, fits most hands. Only a beautiful hand can afford to direct attention to itself by exaggeration of shape and color.

Typists, pianists and other people who perform work with their hands usually require shorter, more rounded-shaped nails in order to avoid nail breakage and injury.

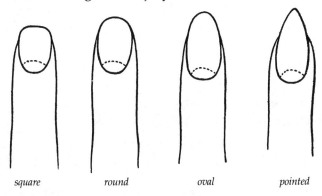

square   *round*   *oval*   *pointed*

PROCEDURE FOR A PLAIN MANICURE

Preparation for Treatment

The routine outlined in this text is one of several ways to give a manicure. Whatever routine your instructor outlines for you, the routine is equally correct.

1. Select and properly arrange required equipment, sanitized instruments, cosmetics and materials.
2. Place clean towel on cushion.
3. Wash manicurist's hands.
4. Pour warm water into finger bowl, to which add a few drops of liquid cleaner and a few drops of antiseptic.
5. Seat client at table and rest the client's arm on cushion.
6. Examine the client's nails.
7. Wipe off tips of fingers with 70% alcohol or appropiate antiseptic.

Procedure

1. Remove old polish. Moisten a pledget with nail polish remover. Using a downward, rotary motion, remove old polish from nails of both hands.

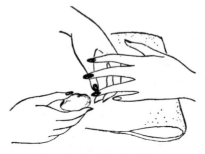

Removing liquid nail polish.

Alternate method of removing nail polish is to moisten small pieces of cotton with nail polish remover and press over old polish on each nail. Then moisten another pledget of cotton with nail polish remover and use for removing the small pledgets on the nails. This acts like a blotter and does not leave a polish smear on cuticle.

With a cotton-tipped orangewood stick dipped in nail polish remover, clean around the cuticle, if necessary.

2. Shape nails. Discuss with client the most suitable nail shape. File the nails of the left hand, from the little finger toward the thumb, in the following manner:

a) Hold the client's finger between the thumb and first two fingers of the left hand.

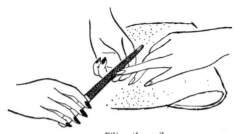

Filing the nails.

b) Hold the file in the right hand and tilt it slightly so that filing is confined mainly to the under side of the free edge.

c) Shape nails into graceful oval tips, never extreme points. Use the coarse side of file or emery board to shape the nail. File each nail from corner to center, going from right to left and then from left to right. On each side of the nail, use two short, quick strokes and one long, sweeping stroke.

Caution: Never file deep into the corners of the nail. If the nails are permitted to grow out at the sides, they will look longer and wear better.

3. Soften cuticle. After completing the left hand, file two nails of the right hand as described above. Then, immerse left hand into finger bowl (cleansing bath) to permit softening of the cuticle. Finish filing nails of right hand. Remove left hand from finger bowl.

4. Dry fingertips. Holding a towel with both hands, carefully dry the left hand, including the area between the fingers. At the same time, gently loosen and push back the cuticle and adhering skin on each nail. Also rub off any dirt deposits present on the nail.

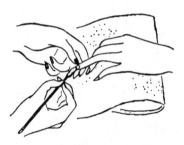

Applying solvent with orangewood stick.

5. Apply cuticle remover (solvent). Wind a thin layer of cotton around the blunt edge of an orangewood stick for use as an applicator. Spread cuticle remover sufficiently over cuticle around nails and under the free edge of left hand.

6. Loosen cuticle. Use the spoon end of the cuticle pusher to gently loosen the cuticle. Keep cuticle moist while working. Use the cuticle pusher in a flat position to remove dead cuticle adhering to the nail without scraching the nail plate. Push cuticle back with towel over index finger.

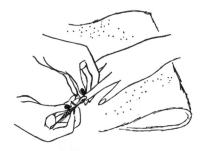

Loosening cuticle with cuticle pusher.

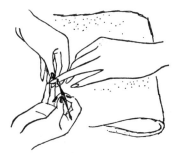

Removing dead cuticle with cuticle pusher.

In using both the cuticle pusher and orangewood stick, avoid too much pressure so that live tissue at the root of the nail will not be injured.

7. Clean under free edge. Use cotton-tipped orangewood stick; dip in soapy water and clean under free edge, from the center toward each side, with gentle pressure.

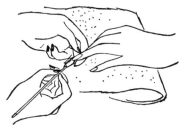

Cleaning under free edge.

8. Trim cuticle. If necessary, use cuticle nippers to remove dead cuticle, hangnails or uneven cuticle. In cutting the cuticle, be careful to remove it as a single segment.

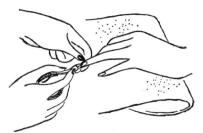

Trim cuticle only where necessary.

9. When cutting the cuticle of the middle finger of the left hand, immerse fingers of the right hand into finger bowl, while continuing to manicure the left hand.

Caution: Be extremely careful to avoid cutting the client's skin. However, be prepared to deal with small cuts by having hydrogen peroxide, powdered alum (styptic powder), or alum solution immediately available.

10. Bleach under free edges with cotton-tipped orangewood stick, if desired. Apply hydrogen peroxide or other bleaching preparation under each free edge of nails of left hand.

Apply nail whitening (optional). Use orangewood stick as applicator, apply chalk paste or string treated with nail whitening under free edge of nails.

11. Apply cuticle oil or cream around the sides and base of the nail and massage with the thumb in a rotary movement.

12. Remove right hand from finger bowl. Treat nails and cuticle of right hand as described under steps 4 to 11.

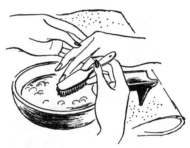

Scrubbing the nails.

13. Cleanse nails. Brush nails in soap bath with a downward movement to remove grease and nail whitening from the nails of both hands.

14. Dry hands and nails thoroughly.

Completion

1. Bevel nails. Carefully re-examine the nails for defects. Use fine side of emery board like a nail file to give the nails a smooth beveled edge. Remove pieces of cuticle.

Buff Nail. Buff nails only if requested by the client. For method of buffing the nails, consult Men's Manicure. To remove powder polish particles before applying base coat, wash and dry the fingers of both hands.

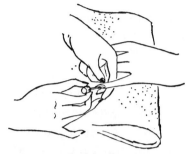

Applying base coat.

Note: As an added service, a hand massage or a hand and arm massage may be given at this time.

2. If required, repair split or broken nails.

3. Apply base coat. Apply base coat with long strokes to the left hand, starting with the little finger to the thumb, then to the right hand, starting with the little finger working toward the thumb. Allow to dry until "slick to a light touch."

4. Apply liquid polish. Dip the camel's-hair brush into the polish and wipe off excess by pressing it gently against the sides of the bottle. Apply the polish lightly and quickly, using sweeping strokes to the free edge of the nail as outlined on the illustrations.

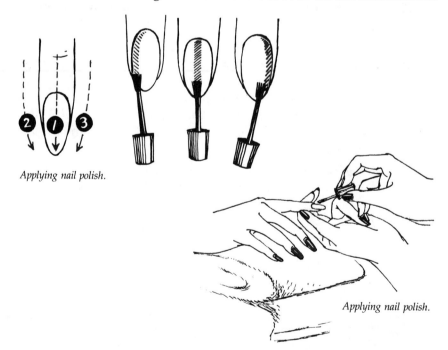

Applying nail polish.

Applying nail polish.

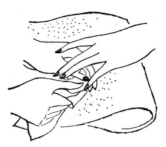

Removing excess polish from tips of nails.

Remove nail polish at hairline tip of nail after each coat of polish. Dip the brush in the polish each time before applying polish to the next nail.

Always keep the polish thin enough to flow freely. If the polish is thick, add a little polish solvent and then shake it well.

5. Remove excess polish. Dip cotton-tipped orangewood stick into nail polish remover. Apply it carefully around the cuticles and nail edges to remove excess polish.

6. Apply top coat or sealer. Apply top coat with long strokes to the left hand and then to the right in the same manner as the base coat. Brush around and under tips of nails for added support and protection.

Note: top coat application is usually eliminated when liquid polish is sprayed with nail enamel dryer.

7. Apply hand lotion. After the top coat is completely dry, as an extra service, apply hand lotion with light manipulations over the hands from wrists to fingertips.

Final Sanitary Care
1. Sanitize used manicure implements and place them in a cabinet sterilizer.
2. Discard used materials (tissues, cotton, etc.) in closed containers.
3. Clean top of manicure table with disinfectant and place everything in order.
4. Clean tops of nail polish bottles with polish remover.
5. Inspect the manicuring table drawer for cleanliness and order.
6. Wash and dry manicurist's hands.

To combine a manicure with a hand and arm massage, see procedure for Hand and Arm Massage.

Individual Nail Styling

Shape of Nails

For a more natural effect, the shape of the nail should conform to that of the fingertip. A gracefully shaped nail adds beauty to the hands.

Nail shapes may be divided into four types:

1. Oval.
2. Slender, tapering (pointed).
3. Square or rectangular.
4. Clubbed (round).

OVAL NAIL

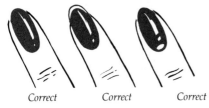

Correct   Correct   Correct

SLENDER, TAPERING (POINTED) NAIL

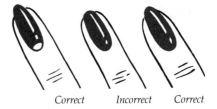

Correct   Incorrect   Correct

The **oval nail** is the ideal nail shape and can be styled either by covering the entire nail with polish, by leaving the free edge white, or by leaving the half moon white at the base of the nail.

The **slender tapering nail** is well suited for the thin, delicate hand. The nail should be tapered somewhat longer than usual to enhance the slender appearance of the hand. The nail can be completely polished, or a half moon can be left at the base.

SQUARE OR RECTANGULAR NAIL

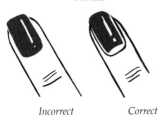

Incorrect   Correct

CLUBBED (ROUND) NAIL

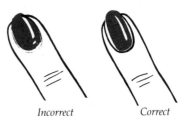

Incorrect   Correct

The **square or rectangular nail** should extend only slightly past the tip of the finger with the nail tip rounded off. The entire nail may be polished with a slight half moon left at the base, and a white margin left at the sides of the nail.

The **clubbed nail** should be slightly tapered and extend just a bit past the tip of the finger. The entire nail should be polished with a thin white margin left at the sides.

Sanitation Rules in Manicuring

The manicurist has the responsibility of sanitizing all manicure implements after each separate use on a client.

To protect the client's welfare, the manicurist should obey the following rules of sanitation.

1. Wear a clean uniform at all times.
2. Wash hands thoroughly before and after each manicure.
3. Use a clean, sanitized towel for each client.
4. Sanitize manicure implements in the following manner:
    a) Wash implements in hot soapy water. Files and nippers should be wiped with alcohol to clear them of particles of nail or skin.
    b) Rinse, then immerse them in a sanitizing solution. The time required depends upon the disinfectant solution used and your state board of cosmetology regulations.
    c) Rinse, dry and place instruments in dry sanitizer until used.
5. Before and during the manicure, place manicure implements in an alcohol wet sanitizer.

Safety Rules in Manicuring

Observing safety rules in manicuring can be of great help in preventing accidents and injury to the client or manicurist. The following safety rules will guide the manicurist in protecting the client.

1. Keep all containers covered and labeled.
2. Use dry hands to hold or move containers.
3. Handle sharp-pointed implements carefully and avoid dropping them.
4. Dull over-sharpened cutting edges of sharp implements with an emery board.
5. Bevel a sharp nail edge with an emery board.
6. Don't file too deeply into nail corners.

7. Avoid excessive friction in nail buffing.

8. Apply an antiseptic immediately if the skin is accidentally cut.

9. Apply styptic powder to stop the bleeding from a small cut. Never use a styptic pencil.

10. Avoid pushing the cuticle back too far.

11. Avoid too much pressure at the base of the nail.

12. Do not use a sharp, pointed instrument to cleanse under the nails.

13. Do not work on a nail when the surrounding skin is inflamed or contains pus.

Oil Manicure

An oil manicure is of particular benefit for ridged and brittle nails and for dry cuticles. It also improves the hands by leaving the skin soft and pliable.

Procedure

1. Heat mineral oil, olive oil or commercial preparation in an electric heater.

2. Proceed with the manicure to the point where you place the hand in the finger bowl; instead, have client place fingers in the heated oil.

3. Massage the hands and wrists with the oil then the cuticles are treated in the usual manner.

4. Wash oil from the hands with warm damp towel.

5. Complete as for a plain manicure.

Men's Manicure

Men usually prefer a conservative manicure. The nails are filed either round or square and a dry polish is applied instead of a liquid polish.

Implements, materials and supplies are the same as those used for a regular manicure. Follow procedure for a general manicure up to the application of base coat.

Buffing the nails.

Buff nails (where permitted). Apply a small amount of powder polish over the buffer. Then buff the nails with 8 to 10 downward strokes from the base to the free edge of each nail. To prevent a heating or burning sensation, lift the buffer from the nail after each stroke. Buffing the nails increases the circulation of the blood to the finger tips, smoothes the nails and gives them a natural gloss or sheen.

If a clear or neutral liquid polish is to be given, remove powder polish particles by washing and drying the finger tips before applying base coat to the nails. Then apply neutral liquid polish and top coat as in the regular manicure.

Booth Manicure

A booth manicure is a timesaver for both client and manicurist. A hurried client may have this type of service when he or she would not have time for a regular table manicure.

A booth manicure is usually given while a client is receiving another service—for example, while a man is having his hair cut or styled.

1. Place implements and supplies in basket lined with a clean, sanitized towel, ready for use.
2. Adjust the manicuring stool at left of client.

When the cosmetologist is working on the left side of the client, the manicurist places stool on right side of client and starts manicure on the right hand.

3. Remove polish from left hand only.
4. Remove polish from right hand. (This is the only time you will have to reach across in front of client.)
5. Remove left hand from soap bath and complete manicure on left hand.
6. Move stool to client's right and complete manicure on right hand.
7. Clean up station, discard used materials, return supplies, sanitize implements and wash hands in the usual manner.

Electric Manicure

The electric manicure is given with the aid of a portable device operated by a small motor. It uses a variety of attachments, which may include an emery wheel, cuticle pusher, cuticle brush and buffer.

Before using an electric manicure machine, read manufacturer's instructions carefully. State regulations on this procedure may vary.

Additional Techniques

A fringe of loose skin left around the nail after a manicure is caused by trimming the cuticle closer than necessary and then rolling back the epidermis. To prevent the occurence of such loose skin, the cuticle should be trimmed only enough to allow a tiny margin of cuticle to remain.

Callous growth at the fingertips can be softened and removed by regular rubbing with the course side of the emery board or with pumice.

To make wide nails appear narrower and longer, apply the lacquer to the nails with a small margin left uncovered at each side.

Stains on fingernails may be bleached with prepared nail bleach, peroxide, or lemon juice. If none of these bleaching treatments are successful, the nail blade may be carefully scraped with an emery board.

Manicure with Hand Massage

A manicure with hand massage is recommended to keep the client's hand looking youthful, firm, well-groomed and smooth.

Equipment Needed

Manicure implements	Hand lotion
Therapeutic lamp	Astringent lotion
Cleansing cream	Cleansing tissue
Massage cream	Emollient cream

General Procedure

1. Rest client's arm on table; expose arms above elbows; lay sanitized towel over shoulder and tuck one end under cuff of sleeve to protect clothing.
2. Remove old nail polish.
3. Apply cleansing cream to hands and wrists.
4. Remove cleansing cream with tissues.
5. Apply emollient cream over hands.
6. Expose hand to heating lamp for five minutes.
7. Give manicure up to the step involving scrubbing the fingers.
8. Apply massage cream to hands.
9. Give hand massage as outlined in steps 1-7 below.
10. Wipe off massage cream with warm steam towel.
11. Apply astringent lotion with cotton.
12. Scrub fingers and nails, and complete manicure.
13. Apply hand lotion.

Procedure for Hand Massage

1. Hold the client's hand in your hand. Place hand lotion on the back of the client's hand and spread it to the fingers and wrist.

2. Hold the client's hand firmly, as in Fig. 1. Bend the hand slowly forward and backward to limber the wrist. Repeat three times.

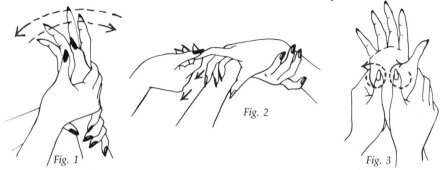

Fig. 1

Fig. 2

Fig. 3

3. Grasp each finger, as in Fig. 2. Gently bend each finger to limber the top of the hand and finger joints. As the fingers and thumb are bent, slide your thumb down toward the fingertips.

4. With the client's elbow resting on the table, hold the hand upright, as in Fig. 3. Massage the palm of the hand with the cushions of your thumbs, using a circular movement in alternate directions. This movement will relax the client's hand.

5. Rest client's arm on the table. Grasp each finger at the base, and rotate it gently in large circles, ending with a gentle squeeze of the fingertips, as in Fig. 4. Repeat three times.

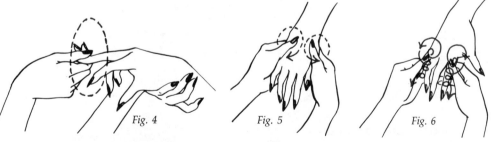

Fig. 4

Fig. 5

Fig. 6

6. Hold the client's hand, as in Fig. 5. Massage wrist, then top of the hand, with a circular movement. Slide back and wring wrist in opposite direction three times. Repeat movements three times.

7. Finish massage by tapering each finger. Begin at base of finger, rotate, pause, and squeeze with gentle pressure. Then, pull lightly with pressure to tip (Fig. 6). Repeat three times.

8. Repeat steps 1 to 7 on other hand.

Manicure with Hand and Arm Massage
The procedure used is similar to manicure with hand massage.
All applications, including massage, are extended to the forearm.

Hand and Arm Massage
1. Complete hand massage as outlined
   previously.

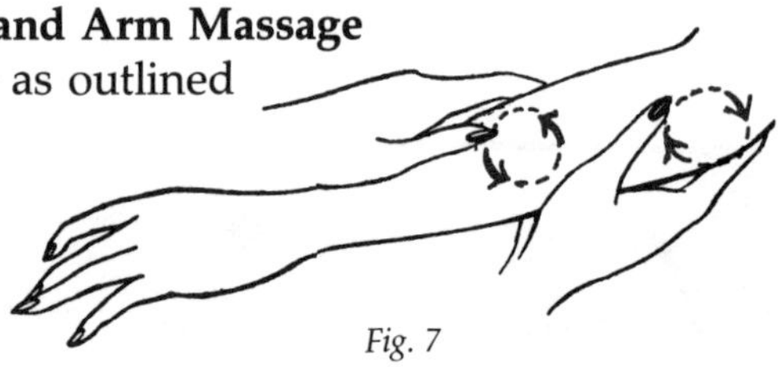

Fig. 7

2. Place client's arm on table, palm
   turned downward as in Fig. 7.
   Massage arms from wrist to elbow.
   Use a slow circular motion in alternate directions. Repeat three times.
   Turn client's arm upwards and
   repeat same movments three times.

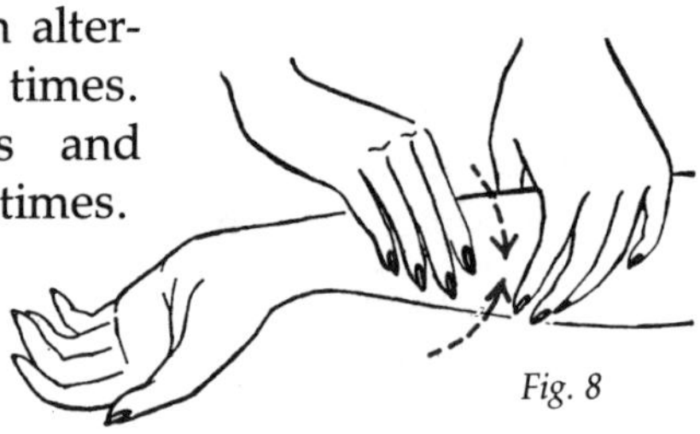

Fig. 8

3. Place your fingers as in Fig. 8.
   Massage deeply under-part of arm to
   the elbow, using fingers of each
   hand in alternate crosswise directions. Repeat three times.

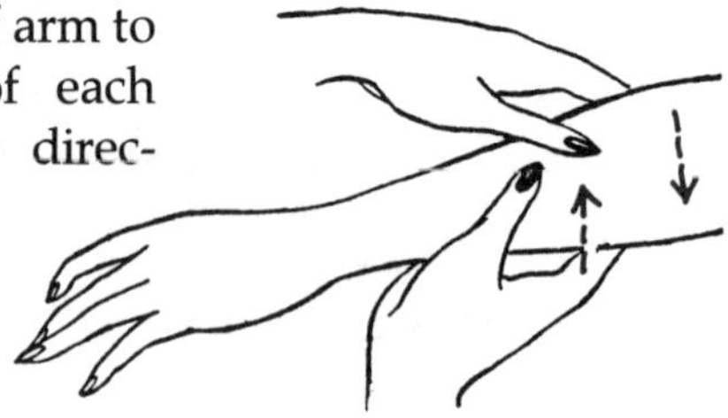

Fig. 9

4. Place your hands as in Fig. 9.
   Massage top of arm. Apply thumbs
   in opposite directions with a squeez-
   ing motion. Repeat three times.

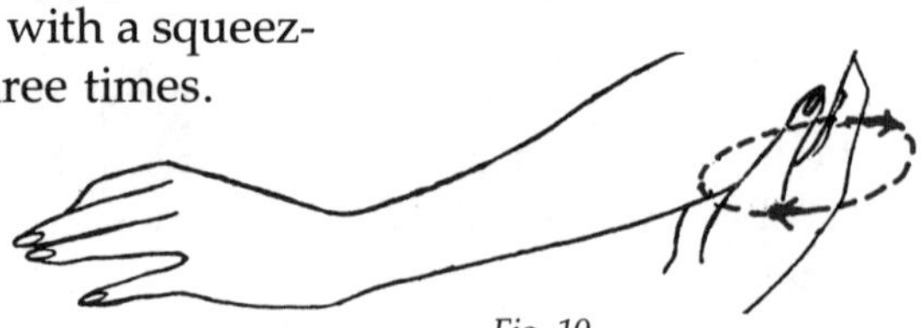

Fig. 10

5. Cup your hand into elbow joint as in Fig. 10. Massage elbow
   with a circular motion. Repeat three times.

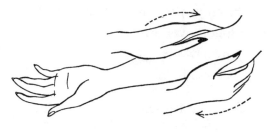

Fig. 11

6. Turn client's palm upwards as in Fig. 11. Stroke arm firmly in opposite directions from the elbow to the wrist. Finally, stroke each finger, ending with a gentle squeeze of the fingertips.

7. Repeat steps 1-6 on other arm.

Hand and Arm Bleach

The purpose of a hand and arm bleach is to lighten a tanned or freckled skin. The bleaching action of the peroxide also lightens the hair on the skin and makes it less noticeable.

Implements and supplies needed for this beauty service include:

Cleansing cream
Cleansing tissues
Astringent lotion
Absorbent cotton
Spatula
Sanitizer
Steam towel

Pillow and safety pins
Commercial bleach cream
or paste
Bleach pase
Ammonia water
(optional). Add 10 drops
to each oz. of bleach
preparation in order to
bleach hair on arms.)
Hydrogen peroxide

Procedure

1. Expose client's entire arms and shoulders.

2. Spread cleansing cream over arms.

3. Remove cleansing cream with tissues.

4. Apply bleach cream or paste over arms, including the elbows, knuckles and fingers.

5. Retain bleach on arms for 10 to 20 minutes, depending on results desired.

6. Prepare steam towel.

7. Remove bleach cream or paste with steam towel.

8. Apply astringent lotion over arms.

9. Dust on talcum powder.

10. Help client to get dressed.

Hand and Arm Bleach Combined with Massage and Manicure

1. Expose client's entire arms and shoulders.

2. Give hand and arm massage.

3. Apply bleach cream or paste over arms.

4. Give manicure up to application or base coat.

5. Prepare steam towel.

6. Remove bleach cream or paste with steam towel.

7. Apply astringent lotion; dust on talcum powder.

8. Complete manicure in the usual manner.

9. Help client to get dressed.

Pedicuring

Pedicuring is the care of the feet, toes, and toenails. It has become an important salon service because the toes and heels in today's shoe fashions are often exposed. Neglected toenails and rough, harsh heels detract from the loveliest of footwear. Foot care not only improves personal appearance, it also adds to the comfort of the feet.

Abnormal foot conditions, such as corns, callouses, and ingrown nails, are best treated by a qualified podiatrist.

Ringworm of the foot (athlete's foot) is an infectious condition which can spread from one person to another. In acute conditions, deeply seated, itchy, colorless vesicles appear. These appear either singly or in groups, and sometimes on only one foot. They spread over the sole and between the toes, sometimes involving the nail

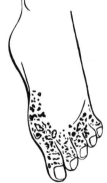

Athlete's foot infection.

fold and infecting the nail. When the vesicles rupture, the skin becomes red and oozes. The lesions dry as they heal. Fungus infection of the feet is likely to become chronic.

The prevention of infection and the treatment of infection are both accomplished by keeping the skin cool, dry, and clean.

CAUTION: Clients with athlete's foot (watery blisters and thick white skin between the toes) or other foot infections should not be given a pedicure. They should be referred to a physician for medical help.

Equipment, Implements, and Materials
The equipment, implements, and materials required for pedicuring are the same as those for manicuring, with the following additions:

Low stool for cosmetologist or pedicurist.

Ottoman on which to rest patron's foot.

Two basins of warm water, each large enough for foot bath and rinse.

Waterproof apron, or an extra towel, to place over the lap to protect the uniform.

Two towels for drying client's feet.

Special toenail clippers.

Witch hazel or other astringent.

Antiseptic solution.

Cotton pledgets and **foot powder.**

Paper towels.

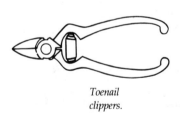

Toenail clippers.

Preparation
1. Arrange required equipment, implements, and materials.
2. Seat client in facial chair; have patron remove shoes and hose.
3. Place his or her feet on a clean paper towel on footrest.
4. Wash your hands.
5. Fill the two basins with enough warm water to cover her ankles.
6. Add antiseptic to one basin. Place both feet in bath for 3-5 minutes.
7. Remove feet from basin, rinse feet in second basin, and wipe dry.

Procedure

1. Remove old polish from the nails of both feet. (Fig. 1)
2. File toenails of the left foot with an emery board. File the toenails straight across, rounding them slightly at the corners to conform to the shape of the toes. To avoid ingrown nails, do not file into the corners of the nails. Smooth rough edges with the fine side of an emery board. (Fig.2)

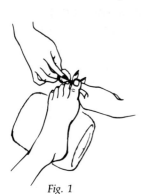

Fig. 1

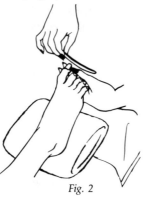

Fig. 2

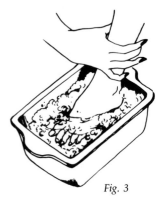

Fig. 3

3. Place the left foot in warm, soapy water (Fig. 3).
4. Shape the nails of the right foot.
5. Remove the left foot from the basin and dry (Fig. 4).
6. With a cotton-tipped orangewood stick, apply cuticle solvent to the cuticle and under the free edge of each toenail (Fig. 5).
7. Place the right foot in the bath.
8. Loosen the cuticle gently on the left foot with a cotton-tipped orangewood stick. Keep the cuticle moist with additional lotion or water. Do not use too much pressure. Avoid the use of the metal pusher.
9. Do not cut the cuticle. Only nip a large, ragged hangnail.
10. Rinse the left foot and dry. Massage each toe with cuticle cream or oil.
11. Repeat steps 5 to 10 on right foot.
12. Scrub both feet in warm, soapy water, rinse, and dry thoroughly.

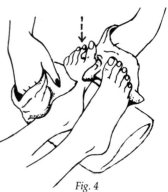

Fig. 4

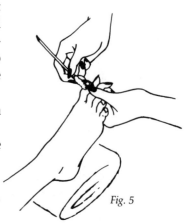

Fig. 5

Foot Massage

1. Apply lotion or cream over the foot to just above the ankle.
2. Start at the instep of the left foot and apply firm, rotary movements down to the center of the toes (Fig. 1).
3. Slide the thumbs firmly back to the instep, and repeat same movement.
4. Slide the thumbs back to the hollow of the heel, and repeat same movement.
5. Slide the thumbs back to the base of the foot, and repeat same movement.
6. Start at the heel and work down to the center of the toes (Fig. 2).
7. Slide firmly back to the heel, and repeat same movement up each side of the foot.

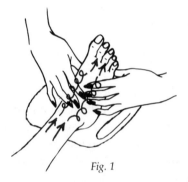

Fig. 1

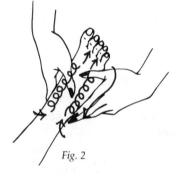

Fig. 2

8. Hold one toe in one hand and the heel in the other hand, and apply three rotary movements; do the same with the other toes (Fig. 3).
9. Slide the right hand to the ankle and the heel of your left hand to the ball of the foot, and apply six firm, rotary movements (Fig. 4).
10. Change to the right foot and repeat Steps 2 to 9.

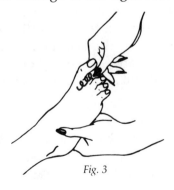

Fig. 3

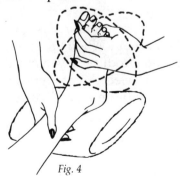

Fig. 4

Completion

1. Remove lotion or cream from both feet with a warm towel.
2. Apply witch hazel or astringent to the feet with a large cotton pledget.
3. Dust lightly with talcum powder.
4. Wipe each toenail with polish remover to remove all traces of lotion or cream.

Note—Inserting cotton between the toes before application of polish will prevent smearing.

5. Apply a base coat, polish, and seal coat in the same manner as for a manicure.
6. Cleanup. Clean and sanitize implements, and place in dry sanitizer. Discard used materials. Clean up the booth. Wash your hands.

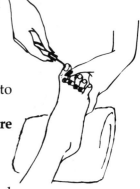
Applying base coat.

Miscellaneous Treatments

Leg Massage

The foot massage may be extended up to and over the knee. When massaging from the ankle to the knee, **do not massage over the shinbone and above the knee.** It is advisable to keep the pressure to the muscular tissue on either side of the shinbone. On the calf area of the leg, you may use kneading upward movements up to the underpart of the knee.

Leg Treatment

To warm the legs in cold weather, briskly rub the leg toward the knee with a finishing cream or lotion.

To cool the legs in warm weather, gently pat or stroke the leg toward the knee with with hazel or another astringent.

Leg Makeup

During warm weather, leg makeup is optional. In addition to a pedicure and foot massage, clients may request the application of leg makeup. When properly applied over legs, this type of makeup should produce a velvety finish without any blotches. For best results, select the proper shade of leg makeup and work quickly according to the manufacturer's directions.

Hiding Varicose Veins

Besides recommending that the client with a bad case of varicose veins consult a doctor, the pedicurist can suggest the use of a waterproof commercial product for concealing varicose veins disfiguration.

MANICURING: A Review

1. **What is meant by manicuring?**	Manicuring is the artful care of the hands and nails.
2. **In what manner does a manicurist prepare the table for a manicure?**	The manicurist selects and arranges sanitary instruments, cosmetics and materials in an orderly manner.
3. **When does the manicurist wash his or her hands for a manicure?**	Before and after each manicure.
4. **When are manicuring implements sanitized?**	Used manicuring implements are sanitized after each manicure.
5. **List five essential implements used in manicuring.**	Nail file, emery boards, cuticle pusher, orangewood sticks and cuticle nippers.
6. **List the most commonly used cosmetics in manicuring.**	Nail polish remover, cuticle solvent, cuticle oil, cuticle cream, nail bleach, nail white, nail polish, base coat and top coat or sealer.
7. **List the important steps in giving a plain manicure.**	Remove old polish; file nails; soften cuticle; appy cuticle solvent; loosen and push back cuticle; trim dead cuticle; cleanse nails and apply base coat, nail polish and top coat.
8. **How often should a manicure be given?**	At least once a week.
9. **Why should filing be done from the corners to the center of the nails?**	Nails are filed with the growth of the nails to avoid splitting.
10. **After an accidental cut in manicuring, what do you apply to avoid an infection?**	Apply an approved antiseptic to prevent infection.
11. **For what purpose is powdered or liquid alum used in manicuring?**	Powdered or liquid alum may be used to stop minor bleeding in manicuring.
12. **What is the action of the cleanser bath?**	To soften the cuticle.
13. **What is the action of a cuticle solvent?**	to soften cuticle and to remove dead cuticle.
14. **Why is a base coat applied before the nail polish?**	Base coat serves as an adhesive base for liquid nail polish.
15. **What is the purpose of the top coat or sealer?**	The top coat or sealer protects the nails from chipping.

16. **For what nail and cuticle conditions is an oil manicure recommended?**

An oil manicure is recommended for brittle nails and dry cuticles.

17. **What is the purpose of hand and arm massage?**

Hand and arm massage increases suppleness and flexibility, improves the texture of the skin, and increases the circulation of the blood to the hand and arms.

PEDICURING: A Review

1. **What is meant by pedicuring?**

Pedicuring is the beautification of the feet and toenails.

2. **Which foot conditions should not be treated by the manicurist?**

Corns, callouses, ingrown nails, foot infections and ringworm of the feet (athlete's foot).

3. **What are the signs of athlete's foot?**

Watery blisters and thick white skin between the toes.

4. **Why should athlete's foot not be treated in a beauty salon?**

It is an infectious condition which can be spread from one person to another.

5. **How can ingrown toenails be prevented in pedicuring?**

File the toenails rounding them slightly to conform to shape of toes. To avoid ingrown nails, do not file or clip into corners of nails.

Advanced Nail Techniques
Artificial Nails

Clean, attractive hands and nails are an admirable part of a woman's top-to-toe grooming. When a woman cannot grow natural nails of the desired strength and length, she may solve the problem by the application of artificial nails.

Extensions of the natural nail may be made by applying an acrylic material, by pressing on an artificial nail or by a combination of the two. Any artificial nail should look natural and allow the natural nail to grow.

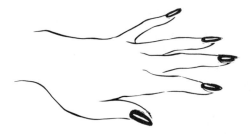

Artificial nails may be used for the following purposes:

1. To conceal broken or damaged nails.
2. To improve the appearance of very short or badly shaped nails.
3. To help overcome the habit of nail biting.
4. To protect a nail or nails against splitting or breakage.

The following techniques will be discussed in this section:

Nail wrapping	Nail tipping
Nail sculpturing	Press-on artificial nails
Fill-in	Nail dipping
Nail capping	Light cured nails

REMINDER

There may be other ways in which the nail techniques presented here are performed. These routines may be changed to meet your instructor's requirements.

Nail Wrapping

Nail wrapping is used to mend torn, broken or split nails, and to fortify weak or fragile nails (Fig. 1). Mending tissue, silk, linen, plastic or liquid fiber are among the materials available for use in this procedure. Bolstering nails with silk will give a smooth, even appearance to the nail. Linen, due to the coarseness of the material, will give a more durable wrap, though a colored polish will be needed to cover the completed nail.

The following two procedures are for use with materials which must be torn to fit the nail or nail fissure. Several manufacturers have recently pre-cut swatches of material which are adhesive backed and are attached *only* to the front of the nail.

CAUTION: Clients should not wear gloves over nails that have been wrapped, as moisture and heat tend to melt the glue and cause bubbles to form under the wrap.

Equipment Needed

Manicuring implements and supplies
Nail adhesive (glue)
Mending tissue
Silk, linen, plastic or liquid fiber

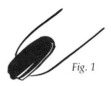

Fig. 1

Procedure for Mending the Nail

1. Lightly file the split or chipped portion of the nail with the fine side of the emery board to help the mending material adhere to the nail.
2. Tear a small piece of mending material and saturate it with the mending adhesive.
3. Place saturated material over the split or chipped area.
4. Tuck the material under the nail with an orangewood stick. The surface of the patch must be smoothed away from the nail edge with an orangewood stick dipped in polish remover.
5. If the split is deep, add a second patch for reinforcement.
6. Dry patch thoroughly before applying the base coat and polish.

Procedure for Fortifying the Nail

1. Give a manicure up to, but not including, the application of the base coat. Scrub the nails to remove oil from the area.

2. Buff the nail surface (Fig. 2).

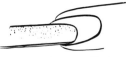
Fig. 2

3. Tear the wrapping material to fit the nail. If using mending tissue, tear it into strips. The tissue or material should be torn so that it is feathered at the edges (Fig. 3).

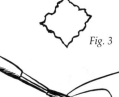
Fig. 3

4. If using mending tissue, saturate each strip with mending adhesive. If using other material, place a line of mending adhesive down the center of the nail (Fig. 4).

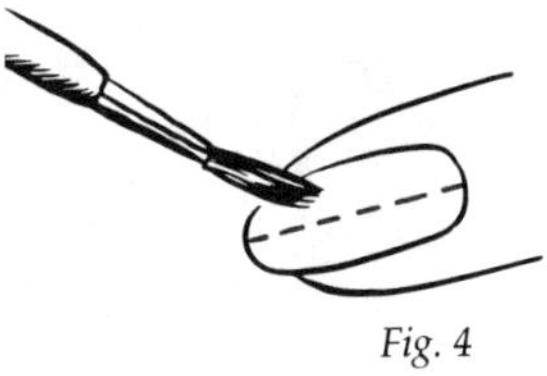

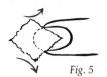
Fig. 4

5. Using two fingers, place the wrapping tissue over the nail. Starting at the middle of the nail, use the pusher to push the tissue in all directions, toward the edges and tip of the nail. Keep dipping the pusher into the remover and patting the tissue until it is smooth (Fig. 5).

Fig. 5

6. Trim excess wrapping tissue extending beyond the free edge and sides of the nail (Fig. 6).

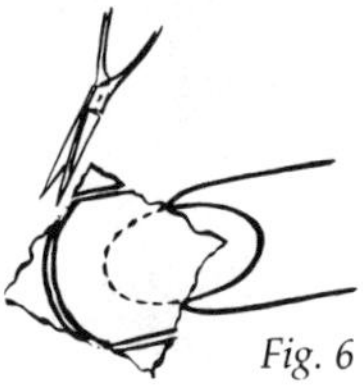

7. Turn the finger over and apply adhesive on the underside of the nail. Then, using the fingertips, fold the tissue over the nail edges.

8. Smooth out the tissue under the free edge with a pusher (Fig. 7).

Fig. 6

9. Repeat steps 2-7 for the other nails.

10. To achieve a smoother finish, gently smooth out the top of the wrapping tissue with the fine side of the emery board. This removes any minute particles that may cause bubbling.

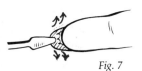
Fig. 7

11. Apply two or three coats of adhesive on the top and underside of the free edge of the nail.

12. Apply a protective base coat on the top and underside of the free edge of the nail, and allow it to dry. Apply nail enamel and top coat or sealer the same as for a regular manicure (Fig. 8).

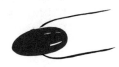
Fig. 8

Alternate Method

In step 4, when applying mending tissue, coat the entire nail plate with adhesive and apply tissue.

How to Remove the Wrapping

Remove polish from the client's right hand. To loosen the nail wrap, have the client place his or her fingertips in polish remover or other solvent recommended by your instructor (Fig. 10).

Fig. 10

After removing the polish from the left hand, have the client remove the right hand from the bowl, and ask him or her to place the fingertips of the left hand in the bowl of polish remover. Gently remove the loosened wrap with an orangewood stick or metal pusher, and then place the fingertips in warm oil. Repeat the same procedure for the left hand.

Liquid Nail Wrap

Liquid nail wrap is a polish made up of tiny fibers designed to strengthen and preserve the natural nail as it grows. It is brushed on to the nail in several directions to create a network which, once hardened, protects the nail. It is similar to nail hardener, though it is of a thicker consistency and contains more fiber.

Nail Sculpturing

Sculpturing *(skulp'cher-ing)* nails involves using high strength acrylic *(a-kril'ik)* materials to increase the nails' thickness and length. It also can be used to repair conditions such as weak, bitten, and torn nails.

Equipment Needed

Sable brush	Nail forms
Liquid	Brush cleaner
Powder	Emery boards
2 small plastic containers	Regular implements used in manicure
	Acrylic nippers

Preparation

Preparation for applying an acrylic sculptured nail involves removing the old polish and giving a manicure up to applying the base coat. A through cleansing with a brush and antiseptic soap will eliminate the possibility of fungus forming under the artificial nail. Nails and surrounding cuticle must be carefully inspected to be sure they are free of cuts or inflammation before the application of nail sculpturing materials.

Procedure

When all the nails are to be done, a working sequence is followed similar to that used in a regular manicure. The following basic steps are applied to one nail:

1. Use the fine side of the emery paper to lightly roughen the nail surface. This not only removes natural oil, it also makes the surface of the nail more adhesive.
2. Using an emery board, file into the corners of the nail so that the nail form will fit properly.
3. Use a piece of cotton or cotton swab to remove the filing particles.
4. Peel a nail form from its paper backing, and using the thumb and index finger of each hand, bend the tip to desired nail shape. The adhesive tabs of the nail form grip the sides of the finger when pressed with the thumb and index finger. Check to see that the form is snug under the free edge and level with the natural nail (Fig. 1).

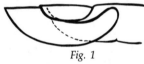

Fig. 1

5. If the product used includes a primer conditioner, it is applied to the surface of the nail at this time with a brush.
6. Pour the liquid and powder components into separate containers. Dip the brush fully into the liquid and wipe once on the edge of the container to remove the excess.
7. Dip the tip of the wet brush into the powder component of the acrylic material, and rotate it slightly as you draw it towards yourself.
8. Place the ball of the acrylic material that forms on the tip of the brush (Fig. 2) on the nail form at the point where the free edge of the natural nail joins the nail form. (Fig. 3).

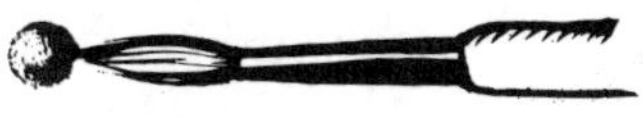

Fig. 2

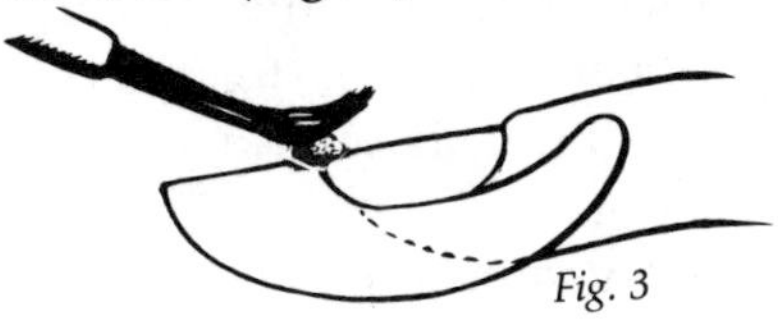

Fig. 3

It is deposited in this position by a slight rotation of the brush. Form the nail by dabbling and pressing the acrylic material into the desired shape at the tip by using the base of the brush (Fig. 4a).

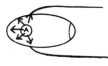

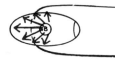

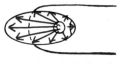

Fig. 4a   *Fig. 4b*   *Fig. 4c*

9. **Second application.** Pick up additional acrylic material as before and place the ball on the nail as indicated in Fig. 4b. Dab and press the material with the brush, working towards the cuticle at the sides of the nail.

10. **Third application.** The third application is the most important for proper retention. Use the mix extremely **wet** (a great deal of liquid and very little powder). Place this mix in the center of the lower half of the nail plate (Fig. 4c). Spread the wet mixture to to the sides. Use caution to avoid contacting the cuticle. Brush excess wet mix onto the body of the nail to smooth out any imperfections.

11. Allow nails to dry thoroughly. Nails are dry when they make a clicking sound when lightly tapped.

12. After the nail has fully hardened, remove the nail form by removing the tabs and pulling downward so that the form detaches.

13. Begin shaping or sculpturing the nail by using a small file at the side of the nail (Fig. 5). Balance the shaping by filing the opposite side as well.

14. Use a large emery board to file the tip and establish the desired length of the nail.

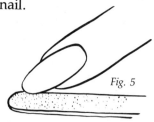

Fig. 5

15. Use the emery board at the sides and on the top of the nail, tapering toward the cuticle and tip.

16. Repeat steps 1-15 for the other nails.

17. Buff the nails with fine emery paper until the entire surface is smooth.

18. Apply cuticle oil, and rub it into the surrounding skin and nail surface.

19. Brush the nails with antiseptic soap to remove debris.
20. Dry the nails thoroughly.
21. Apply the base coat and nail polish or clear nail glaze and top coat, the same as for a regular manicure.

Removing Sculptured Nails

Soak nails in an approved solvent specified by the manufacturer of the nails or recommended by your instructor. When acrylic nails are sufficiently softened, remove them with acrylic nippers using a rolling technique. *DO NOT PRY THE ACRYLIC MATERIAL FROM THE NATURAL NAIL.*

Safety Precautions for Sculptured Nails

1. Clean brush by dipping it into polish remover and wiping it clean.
2. Clean mixing dish by lifting hardened content out with pusher.
3. Make sure bottles are tightly capped when not in use.
4. Do not store product near heat, or use near open flame.
5. Do not apply to injured or inflamed skin.
6. A change in the color of the natural nail after sculptured nails have been applied usually means that fungus is growing under the acrylic. Most primers have aseptic ingredients that sanitize the nail before acrylic is applied. To help ensure that contamination does not occur, *DO NOT TOUCH THE NAIL AFTER THE PRIMER IS APPLIED.*

When sculptured nails lift, crack, or grow out and are not attended to immediately, moisture and dirt become trapped under the acrylic and fungus begins to grow. The spread of fungus can lead to nail injury or loss. Do not attempt to treat the condition yourself. It is very contagious, and the client should be referred to a physician.

Fill-In

As the natural nail grows, it must be filled in after it has grown about 1/8 inch from the cuticle to the edge of the original acrylic on the nail (Fig. 1). Normally a nail grows approximately 1/8 inch a month. In most cases, a fill-in will be needed in about three to four weeks.

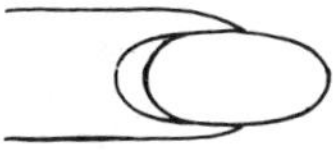

Fig. 1

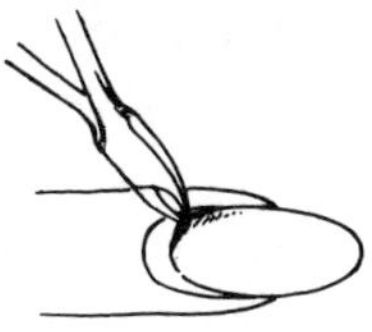

Fig. 2

1. Remove polish and give a thorough cleansing with a brush and antiseptic soap.
2. With nail nippers, clip away loose part of the sculptured nail (Fig. 2). Do not forcibly remove the old acrylic material, but make certain that any loose material is removed. (Reminder: Be careful not to dig into the natural nail. It is best to wear glasses when doing this, as the chips may fly.)
3. With a fine emery board, lightly buff the exposed natural nail surface.
4. Repeat steps 5-21 as outlined on pages 67 and 69.

Nail Capping

Nail capping can strengthen weak nails or repair damaged nails. The acrylic material is used in the same manner as in nail sculpturing, with the following exception:

The nail or nails are not extended but are simply reinforced on the top surface.

Equipment Needed

All the usual materials for nail sculpturing are needed with the exception of nail forms, as the nail tip is not to be extended.

Procedure

The same as in nail sculpturing.

Nail Tipping

Any woman can have long looking nails by simply extending the natural nail artificially.

Procedure

1. Give manicure up to but not including polish.
2. Select proper sized tip to fit client's natural nail (Fig. 1).
3. Slightly roughen the free edge of the nail.
4. File tip to fit the shape of the free edge of the nail only (Fig. 2).
5. Hold nail tip with thumb and index finger and apply half a drop of glue to the free edge of the nail (Fig. 3).
6. Using an orangewod stick, press tip onto the free edge of the nail, and then hold until dry (Fig. 4).
7. Buff the nail where the free edge of the nail and the tip form a seam. Leave resulting dust on nail (Fig. 5).

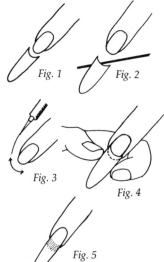

Fig. 1

Fig. 2

Fig. 3

Fig. 4

Fig. 5

8. Apply nail glue to seam where nail tip and free edge of nail meet (Fig. 6). Glue placed over the nail dust will act as a bond and filler. Repeat glue application twice.

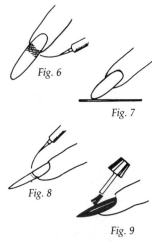

Fig. 6

Fig. 7

9. File sides of tip to blend with the natural nail. Cut nail to desired shape (Fig. 7).
10. Apply glue from seam to the free edge of nail tip (Fig. 8). Buff seam and repeat procedure.
11. Apply nail polish as in a regular manicure (Fig. 9).

Fig. 8

Fig. 9

Removing Nail Tips

To remove nail tips, fill a small container with adhesive solvent recommended by the manufacturer or by your instructor. Soak nail tips until softened (Fig. 10).

Fig. 10

Press-on Artificial Nails

Models, actresses, saleswomen and other women whose hands are on display may wear a complete set of press-on artificial nails every day. Women who do other types of work where their hands are not on display may wish to wear artificial nails only for special occasions.

Artificial nails are constructed of either plastic or nylon, and manufacturer's instructions must be followed carefully. Manufacturers advise against wearing artificial nails for more than 2 weeks to allow for natural nail growth.

Equipment Needed

Regular manicuring implements and materials
Artificial nails
Nail adhesive
Adhesive remover

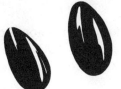

Preparation

1. Remove polish from nails, and give a manicure up to, but not including, the application of polish.
2. Buff the client's nails by going over them with an emery board.
3. Select the proper nail size for each finger. With a sharp manicuring scissors, trim and then file the artificial nail at the cuticle end so that it fits to the shape of the natural nail. Artificial nails can be flattened by being firmly pressed down before application. They also can be reshaped by being held in warm water for a few seconds and molded to the desired shape.

Procedure

1. Apply a small amount of adhesive evenly on the edges of the client's nails. Do not apply adhesive to the center of the nails.
2. Apply adhesive on the inside of the artificial nail, excluding tip.
3. Allow the adhesive to dry throughly (about 2 minutes).
4. Press artificial nail gently onto the natural nail, with the base touching the cuticle or under it. As each nail is applied, hold it firmly in place for about a minute.
5. Carefully wipe away any excess adhesive from tips and around nails.
6. Allow the artificial nails to dry thoroughly. Advise the client to avoid disturbing the nails while they are drying.
7. Finish the manicure by applying base coat, polish, and top coat.

Removing Polish

To remove nail polish from nails constructed of **plastic,** use only nail polish remover that has an oily base and does not contain acetone.

Reminder: Polish remover containing acetone will damage plastic artificial nails.

If **nylon**-constructed fingernails have been used, an acetone type of polish remover will not affect them.

Removing Press-on Artificial Nails

Apply a few drops of oily nail polish remover around the edge of the nail; then gently lift from the side with an orangewood stick.

Do not attempt to pull or twist off the nail, as this could damage or injure the natural nail. Adhesive remover can be used to assist nail remover. It also can be used to remove any surplus adhesive from artificial nails and from natural nails. Artificial nails should be dried carefully and stored in a box. With proper care, they can be reused.

Reminders and Hints on Press-on Artificial Nails

1. Never apply artificial nails over sore or infected areas.
2. Most manufacturers suggest that artificial nails not be worn for more than 2 weeks at a time, in order to allow for natural growth of the nail.
3. Most artificial nail adhesives are flammable, so be cautious with cigarettes, matches, and lighters.
4. When wearing artificial nails, do not subject them to a long period of immersion in water as they might tend to loosen.
5. Do not contaminate the adhesive with oil, cream, or powder.

Nail Dipping

Nail dipping is another method used to extend the nail, utilizing both an acrylic powder and nail tips.

Procedure

1. Remove polish from nails.
2. Sanitize nail with an antibacterial solution.
3. Buff surface of nail to remove excess oil and residue.
4. Apply nail tip, filing sides of tip to fit the free edge of the natural nail.
5. Re-sanitize nail.
6. Apply a thick adhesive coating over the entire surface of the nail, being careful to avoid the cuticle.
7. While adhesive is still wet, slowly insert nail into an acrylic dipping powder. After five seconds, remove nail.
8. When nail dries, remove excess powder from nail surface and lightly file to remove graininess. Be careful not to overfile nail.
9. Seal nail with a thin adhesive.
10. Buff nail until smooth.
11. Cleanse nails with soap and water and polish as in a regular manicure. Repeat entire procedure on remaining nails.

Removal of Dipped Nails

Soak nails until softened in adhesive solvent recommended by the manufacturer or by your instructor.

Light Cured Nails

A method of nail extension in which an acrylic gel is brushed (much like nail polish) onto the nail, either over a nail tip or over a nail form. The nail is then placed under an ultra-violet lamp to dry (utilizing UVA, long wavelength rays). Drying time is usually less than one minute.

Caution should be used when giving this service, as inadequately shielded UVA lamps can cause damage to the eyes and skin.

Nails are removed by softening them in a manufacturer recommended gel remover and then buffing until all acrylic is removed from the nail.

ARTIFICIAL NAILS: A Review

1. **List the important steps in mending the nail with a nail wrap.**	Lightly file nail split or chip. Tear piece of mending material and saturate with adhesive. Place material over split or chip. Tuck material under nail. Smooth with orangewood stick dipped in polish remover.
2. **List the important steps in fortifying the nail with a nail wrap.**	Roughen nail surface with emery board. Tear wrapping material to fit nail. Saturate tissue with adhesive. If using other material, place adhesive down center of nail. Place wrapping material over nail. Trim excess material. Put adhesive on underside of nail. Fold tissue over nail edge. Apply adhesive to top and underside of nail.
3. **What is a liquid nail wrap?**	A liquid nail wrap is a polish made up of tiny fibers that strengthen and preserve the natural nail.
4. **Describe the procedure for removing a nail wrap.**	Remove polish from client's hand. Place fingertips in bowl of polish remover or other solvent. Remove loosened wrap with an orangewood stick or metal pusher. Place fingertips in warm oil.

5. List the important steps in giving a sculptured nail.

1) Give manicure up to but not including hand and arm massage.
2) Roughen nail with emery board
3) Dust nail bed
4) Apply nail primer
5) Peel nail form from its backing and bend to shape.
6) Dip brush into liquid mixture and then into acrylic powder.
7) Place ball on free edge of nail and press to shape.
8) Place additional acrylic material at center of nail and shape.
9) Place wet acrylic mixture on lower half of nail and shape.
10) Let nails dry, remove nail forms
11) File new nails to shape and buff.
12) Wash nail or nails.

6. List the equipment needed for nail sculpturing.

Sable brush, liquid, powder, 2 small plastic containers, nail forms, brush cleaner, emery boards, manicuring implements, acrylic nippers.

7. Why should nails be sanitized before applying acrylic material?

To prevent the growth of fungus.

8. Explain the technique for removing sculptured nails.

Soak nails in solvent. When acrylic is sufficiently softened, remove with acrylic nippers using a rolling technique.

9. When is a fill-in usually needed?

Every three to four weeks.

10. How does nail capping differ from nail sculpturing?

The nail or nails are not extended but are simply reinforced on the top surface.

11. List the steps for nail tipping.

Select tip. Slightly roughen free edge of nail. File tip to fit free edge. Apply glue to free edge. Press tip to free edge. Hold with orangewood stick until dry. Buff nail at point where free edge and tip meet. Apply adhesive to resulting seam twice. Cut and file nail to shape. Apply glue to nail tip, buff, reapply glue. Apply polish.

12. **Explain the procedure for press-on nails.**	Apply adhesive to edge of client's nail. Apply adhesive to inside of artificial nail, excluding tip. Let adhesive dry. Press artificial nail gently to natural nail. Hold in place one minute. Wipe away excess adhesive. Apply base coat, polish and top coat.
13. **What are artificial nails constructed of?**	Plastic or nylon.
14. **What is the maximum time press-on nails can be left on?**	Two Weeks
15. **What should you use to remove nail polish from press-on nails?**	Oily, non-acetone, remover.
16. **List the steps for nail dipping.**	Remove polish, sanitize nail. Buff nail. Apply nail tip. Resanitize nail. Apply thick adhesive, coating entire nail surface. Insert nail into acrylic dipping powder. Remove nail after five seconds. When nail dries, remove excess powder and lightly file nail. Seal nail with thin adhesive. Buff nail. Cleanse nail with soap and water. Apply polish.

Nail Disorders

Diseases of the nail should never be treated by a manicurist. However, the manicurist should recognize normal and abnormal nail conditions, and understand the reasons for these conditions. Simple nail irregularities and blemishes come within the province of cosmetology and can be treated by the manicurist. A client having a nail condition where infection, soreness, or irritation is present should be referred to a physician.

Nail Irregularities

Corrugations, or **wavy ridges,** are caused by uneven growth of the nails, usually the result of illness or injury. When giving a manicure to a client with this condition, carefully buff the nails slightly with pumice powder. This will help to remove or minimize the ridges.

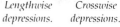

Furrows.

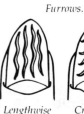

Furrows (depressions) in the nails may run either lengthwise or across the nail. These are usually the result of illness or an injury to the nail cells in or near the matrix. Since these nails are exceedingly fragile, great care must be exercised in giving a manicure. Avoid the use of the metal pusher; use a cotton-tipped orangewood stick around the cuticle.

Lengthwise depressions. *Crosswise depressions.*

Leuconychia *(loo-ko-nik'e-a),* or **white spots,** appear frequently in the nails, but do not indicate disease. They may be caused by injury to the base of the nail. As the nail continues to grow, these white spots eventually disappear.

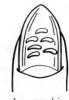

Leuconychia.

Onychauxis *(on-e-kawk'sis),* or **hypertrophy** *(hy-per'tro-fee),* is an over-growth of the nail, usually in thickness rather than length. It is usually caused by an internal disturbance, such as a local infection. If infection is present, the nail is not to be manicured. If infection is not present, the nail may be included in the manicure. File it smooth and buff with pumice powder.

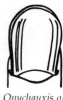

Onychauxis or hypertrophy.

Onychatrophia *(o-nik-a-tro'fee-a),* **atrophy,** or **wasting away,** of the nail causes the nail to lose its luster, become smaller, and sometimes shed entirely. Injury or disease may account for this nail irregularity. File the nail smooth with the fine side of the emery board. Advise the client to protect it from further injury or from exposure to strong soaps and washing powders.

Onychatrophia.

Pterygium *(te-rij'ee-um)* is a forward growth of the cuticle that adheres to the base of the nail. Use the cuticle nippers carefully to remove the growth. Suggest oil manicures.

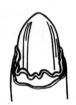

Pterygium.

Onychophagy *(on-e-ko-fay'jee),* or **bitten nails,** is a result of an acquired nervous habit that prompts the individual to chew the nail or the hardened cuticle. Advise the client that frequent manicures and care of hardened cuticle often help to overcome this habit.

Onychophagy.

Onychorrhexis *(on-e-ko-rek'sis)* refers to **split** or **brittle nails.** Among the causes of split nails are injury to the finger, careless filing of the nails, and excessive use of cuticle solvents and nail polish removers. Suggest oil manicures.

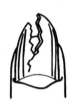

Onychorrhesis.

Hangnail *(agnail)* is a condition in which the cuticle splits around the nail. Dryness of the cuticle, cutting off too much cuticle, or carelessness in removing the cuticle may result in hangnails. Advise the client that proper nail care, such as hot oil manicures, will aid in correcting this condition. If not properly cared for, a hangnail may become infected.

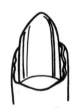

Hangnails.

Eggshell nails are recognized by the nail plate being noticeably thin, white, and much more flexible than normal nails. The nail plate separates from the nail bed and curves at the free edge. This disorder may be caused by a chronic illness of systemic or nervous origin.

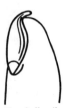

Eggshell nail.

Blue nails may be attributed to poor blood circulation or a heart disorder. However, a client with these conditions may receive a regular manicure.

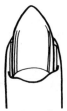

Blue nail.

A **bruised nail** will show dark, purplish (almost black or brown) spots in the nail. These are usually due to injury and bleeding in the nail bed. The dried blood attaches itself to the nail and grows out with it. Treat this injured nail gently. Avoid pressure.

Treating cuts. If a cut is accidentally inflicted on a client during a manicure, apply an antiseptic immediately. Do not buff or apply nail polish to the injured finger. To protect against infection, apply a sterile band-aid.

Infected finger. In the case of an infected finger, the client should be referred to a physician.

Nail Diseases

There are several nail diseases that may be met during cosmetology practice. However, any nail disease that shows signs of infection or inflammation (redness, pain, swelling, or pus) *must not* be treated in a beauty salon. Medical treatment is required for all nail diseases.

Occupation plays an important role in the cause of many nail infections. Infections develop more readily in those who constantly immerse their hands in alkaline solutions. Natural oils are removed from the skin by frequent exposure to soaps, solvents, and other substances. The hands of the cosmetologist are exposed daily to chemical materials. Many of these are harmless, but others have potential dangers. The cosmetologist should safeguard his or her hands and nails by wearing protective gloves when working with chemicals.

Onychosis *(on-i-ko'sis)* is a technical term applied to any nail disease.

Onychomycosis *(on-e-ko-mi-ko'sis)*, **tinea unguium** *(tin'ee-a ung'gwe-um)*, or **ringworm of the nails,** is an infectious disease caused by a vegetable parasite. A common form consists of whitish patches that can be scraped off the surface. Another form appears as long yellowish streaks within the nail substance.

Onychomycosis.

The disease invades the free edge and spreads toward the root. The infected portion is thick and discolored. In a third form, the deeper layers of the nail are invaded, causing the superficial layers to appear irregularly thin. These infected layers peel off and expose the diseased parts of the nail bed.

Ringworm *(tinea)* of the hands is a highly contagious disease caused by a fungus (vegetable parasite). The principal symptoms are papular, red lesions occurring in patches or rings over the hands. Itching may be slight or severe.

Most cases of dermatitis of the hands resemble tinea, but are actually a contact dermatitis, plus a staphylococcic infection. Only a physician can diagnose this condition.

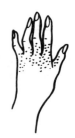

Tinea unguium.

Ringworm of the foot (athlete's foot). In acute conditions, deep, itchy, colorless vesicles appear. These appear singly, in groups, and sometimes on only one foot. They spread over the sole and between the toes, perhaps involving the nail fold and infecting the nail. When the vesicles rupture, the skin becomes red and oozes. The lesions dry as they heal. Fungus infection of the feet is likely to become chronic.

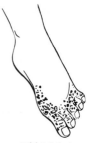

Athlete's foot.

Both the prevention of infection and beneficial treatment are accomplished by keeping the skin cool, dry, and clean.

Paronychia *(par-o-nik'ee-a)*, or **felon,** is an infectious and inflammatory condition of the tissues surrounding the nails. This condition is traceable to bacterial infection.

Onychia is an inflammation of the nail matrix, accompanied by pus formation. Improper sanitization of nail implements and bacterial infection may cause this disease.

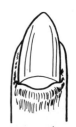

Paronychia.

Onychocryptosis *(on-ik-o-krip-to'sis)*, or **ingrown nails,** may affect either the finger or toe. In this condition, the nail grows into the sides of the flesh and may cause an infection. Filing the nails too much in the corners and failing to correct hangnails are often responsible for ingrown nails.

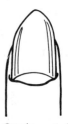

Onychocryptosis.

Onychoptosis *(on-e-kop-to'sis)* is the periodic shedding of one or more nails, either in whole or in part. This condition may follow certain diseases, such as syphilis.

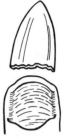

Onychoptosis.

Onycholysis *(on-e-kol'i-sis)* is a loosening of the nail, without shedding. It is frequently associated with an internal disorder.

Onycholysis.

Onychophyma *(on-e-ko-fy'mah)* denotes a swelling of the nail.

Onychophosis *(on-e-ko-fo'sis)* refers to a growth of horny epithelium in the nail bed.

Onychogryposis *(on-e-ko-gri-po'sis)* pertains to enlarged and increased curvature of the nails.

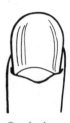

Onychophyma.

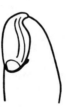

Onychogryposis.

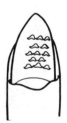

Onychophosis.

NAIL DISORDERS: A Review

1. Should an infected fingernail be given a manicure?	No. The client should be referred to a physician.
2. What may cause wavy ridges?	Uneven growth of the nails, usually the result of illness.
3. List 12 abnormal conditions of the nails that do not prohibit a manicure.	corrugations, furrows, white spots, hypertrophy, atrophy, pterygium, bitten nails, brittle nails, hangnails, eggshell nails, blue nails, bruised nails.
4. What is the technical name for split or brittle nails?	Onychorrhexis.
5. What treatment should you recommend for brittle nails?	Oil manicures.
6. What are hangnails? Give their cause.	Hangnail is a condition in which the cuticle splits around the nail. Dryness of the cuticle, cutting too much cuticle, or carlessness in removing the cuticle may cause hangnails.
7. How are hangnails treated?	With proper nail care, such as a hot oil treatment.
8. How is an accidental cut treated during a manicure?	An antiseptic is applied.
9. Define Onychosis.	Onychosis is a technical term for any nail disease.
10. What parasite causes ringworm?	A vegetable parasite.
11. What are the signs of athlete's foot (ringworm of the foot)?	Deep, itchy, colorless vesicles appear.
12. What causes a paronychia condition?	A bacterial infection.
13. Define Onychia.	Onychia is an inflammation of the nail matrix, accompanied by pus formation.
14. How is paronychia identified?	By an inflammatory condition of the tissues surrounding the toenails.
15. What is the technical term for ingrown nails?	Onychocryptosis.

Anatomy and Physiology

Anatomy *(a-nat'o-mee)* **and physiology** *(fiz-ee-ol'o-jee)* are subjects of considerable importance to the practice of manicuring. Knowledge of the structure and functions of the human body forms the scientific basis for the proper application of beauty treatments. A basic understanding of these subjects will help to improve the professional skill of the manicurist. He or she will then know which manicuring treatment is best for the client's condition and how to adjust and control the treatment for best results.

Anatomy is the study of the client's structure and organs of the body, such as muscles, bones and arteries. The manicurist is concerned only with those parts treated, such as the arms and hands.

Histology *(his-tol'o-jee)* **or microscopic** *(my-kro-skop'ik)* **anatomy** is the study of the minute *(my-nyut')* structure of the various parts of the body. The manicurist is particularly concerned with the histology of the skin and its appendages (nails, hair, sweat and oil glands).

Physiology is the study of the functions or activities performed by the various parts of the body.

ANATOMY AND PHYSIOLOGY: A Review

1. **Why should manicurists study the anatomy of the arms and hands?**	In order to have a constructive knowledge of parts of the body treated during manicure.
2. **Define anatomy.**	Anatomy is the study of the structure and organs of the body, such as muscles, bones or arteries.
3. **Define physiology.**	Physiology is the study of the functions or activities performed by various parts of the body.
4. **Define histology. The manicurist is concerned with the histology of which parts of the body?**	Histology is the study of the minute structure of the body. The manicurist is concerned with the histology of the skin, nails, hair, sweat glands and oil glands.

CELLS

In order to understand anatomy and physiology it is necessary to study the structure and activities of cells. The human body is composed of millions of specialized cells which perform the functions required for living. In giving manicuring treatments, the manicurist should keep in mind the ultimate effect of the treatment on the cells of the body.

Cells are the basic units of all living things, which include humans, animals, plants, and bacteria. Every part of the body is composed of cells, which differ from each other in size, shape, structure, and function.

A cell is a minute portion of living substance containing **protoplasm** (pro'to-plazm), which is a colorless, jelly-like substance in which food elements and water are present. The two main parts of the cell are the **nucleus** and the **cytoplasm.**

Structure of the Cell

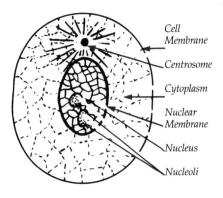

Cell Membrane

Centrosome

Cytoplasm

Nuclear Membrane

Nucleus

Nucleoli

The cell consists of protoplasm and contains the above essential parts.

The protoplasm of the cells contains the following important structures:

Nucleus (dense protoplasm)— found in the center, which plays an important part in the reproduction of the cell.

Cytoplasm (less dense protoplasm)—found outside of the nucleus and contains food materials necessary for the growth, reproduction, and self-repair of the cell.

Centrosome (sen'tro-sohm)— a small, round body in the cytoplasm, which also affects the reproduction of the cell.

Cell membrane encloses the protoplasm. It permits soluble substances to enter and leave the cell.

Cell Growth and Reproduction

As long as the cell receives an adequate supply of food, oxygen and water, eliminates waste products, and is favored with proper temperature, it will continue to grow and thrive. However, if these requirements are not fulfilled, and the presence of toxins (poisons) or pressure is evident, then the growth and the health of the cells are impaired. Most body cells are capable of growth and self-repair during their life cycle.

In the human body, when a cell reaches maturity, reproduction takes place by indirect division. This is a process in which a series of changes occur in the nucleus before the entire cell divides in half. Remember that the nucleus is surrounded by a thinner form of protoplasm, called cytoplasm, which supplies the food materials necessary for growth and reproduction.

Diagram Illustrating Indirect Division of the Human Cell

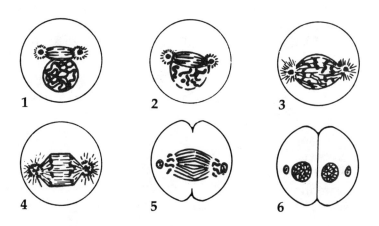

Metabolism

Metabolism *(me-tab'o-lizm)* is a complex chemical process whereby the body cells are nourished and supplied with the energy needed to carry on their many activities.

There are two phases to metabolism:

1. **Anabolism** *(an-ab'o-lizm)* — the building up of cellular tissues. During anabolism, the cells of the body absorb water, food, and oxygen for the purpose of growth, reproduction, and repair.

2. **Catabolism** *(ka-tab'o-lizm)* — the breaking down of cellular tissues. During catabolism, the cells consume what they have absorbed in order to perform specialized functions, such as muscular effort, secretions, or digestion.

Cells have various duties. They create and renew all parts of the body; they assist in blood circulation by carrying food to the blood and waste matter from the blood; and they control all body functions.

THE SKIN

The scientific study of the skin forms the basis for an effective program of skin care and beauty treatments. The skin is the largest organ in the body and performs many vital functions required for health and beauty. The manicurist who has a thorough understanding of the skin, its structure and functions, will be in a better position to give her clients professional advice.

A healthy skin is slightly moist, soft, flexible, slightly acid, and is free from any blemish or disease. Its texture, as revealed by feel and appearance, should be smooth and fine grained. A good complexion shows itself in the fine texture and healthy color of the skin.

The skin varies in thickness, being thinnest on the eyelids and thickest on the palms and soles. Continued pressure over any part of the skin will cause it to thicken, as in a callous.

Histology of the Skin

The skin contains two clearly defined divisions:

1. The **epidermis** *(ep-i-der'mis)*, commonly known as **cuticle** *(kyu'ti-kl)* or **scarf skin,** is the outermost protective layer.

2. The **dermis** *(der'mis)*, also called **derma corium** *(ko'ree-um)*, **cutis** *(kyu'tis)* or **true skin,** is the deeper layer of the skin.

Subcutaneous tissue, also called **adipose tissue** or **subcutis,** is a fatty tissue found below the dermis.*

The **epidermis** or **cuticle** forms the outer protective covering of the skin of the body. It contains no blood vessels but has many small nerve endings. The epidermis contains the following layers:

1. The **stratum corneum** *(strah'tum kor'nee-um)* (horny layer) consists of tightly packed, scale-like cells which are continually being shed and replaced. As these cells develop from underneath layers, they form keratin *(ker'a-tin)*, which acts as a waterproof covering for the skin.

2. The **stratum lucidum** *(loo'si-dum)* (clear layer) consists of small transparent cells through which light can pass.

*Some histologists refer to the subcutaneous tissue as a continuation of the dermis, while others consider it a separate layer.

One Square Inch of Skin Contains:

19,500 sensory cells
at the ends
of nerve fibers

65 hairs

13 sensory
apparatuses for cold

78 sensory apparatuses
for heat

78 yards of
nerves

95-100 sebaceous
glands

19-20 yards of
blood vessels

1,300 nerve endings to
record pain

160-165 pressure apparatuses
for the perception of
tactile stimuli

650 sweat glands

9,500,000 cells

Diagram of a Section of the Scalp

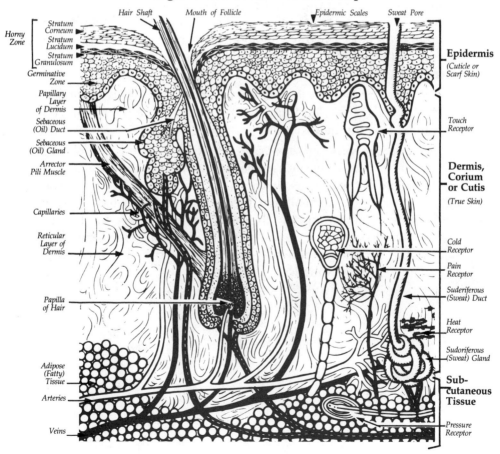

Hair Shaft   Mouth of Follicle   Epidermic Scales   Sweat Pore

Horny Zone

Stratum Corneum
Stratum Lucidum
Stratum Granulosum

Germinative Zone

Papillary Layer of Dermis

Sebaceous (Oil) Duct

Sebaceous (Oil) Gland

Arrector Pili Muscle

Capillaries

Reticular Layer of Dermis

Papilla of Hair

Adipose (Fatty) Tissue

Arteries

Veins

Epidermis
(Cuticle or Scarf Skin)

Touch Receptor

Dermis, Corium or Cutis
(True Skin)

Cold Receptor

Pain Receptor

Suderiferous (Sweat) Duct

Heat Receptor

Sudoriferous (Sweat) Gland

Sub-cutaneous Tissue

Pressure Receptor

3. The **stratum granulosum** *(gran-u-lo'sum)* (granular layer) consists of cells which look like distinct granules. These cells are almost dead and undergo a change into a horny substance.

4. The **stratum germinativum** *(jer'mi-na-tye'vum)*, formerly known as the **stratum mucosum*** *(mew-ko'sum)*, is composed of several layers of differently shaped cells. The deepest layer is responsible for the growth of the epidermis. It also contains a dark skin pigment, called **melanin** *(mel'a-nin)*, which protects the sensitive cells below from the destructive effects of excessive ultraviolet rays of the sun or of an ultraviolet lamp.

The **dermis** is the true skin. It is also called **derma, corium** or **cutis.** In this layer is found an elastic network of cells through which are distributed blood and lymph vessels, nerves, sweat glands and oil glands. It contains the following layers:

1. **The papillary** *(pap'i-ler-ee)* **layer,** which lies directly beneath the epidermis, contains the papillae, or little cone-like projections, made of fine strands of elastic tissue which extend upward into the epidermis. Some of these papillae contain looped capillaries, others contain looped terminations of nerve fibers called **tactile corpuscles** *(tak'til kor'pus-ls)*. This layer also contains some of the **melanin** skin pigment.

2. **The reticular** *(re-tik'yoo-ler)* **layer,** in whose network is contained the fat cells, the blood and lymph vessels, the sweat and oil glands, and the hair follicles.

The **subcutaneous** *(sub-kew-ta'nee-us)* **tissue** (subcutis) *(sub-ku'tis)* or adipose *(ad'i-poce)* tissue is regarded by some histologists as a continuation of the dermis. It varies in thickness according to the age, sex and general health of the individual. This tissue gives smoothness and contour to the body, contains fats for use as energy and also acts as a protective cushion for the outer skin. This fatty tissue contains a network of arteries, and a superficial and deep network of lymphatics.

---

* *Stratum germinativum also is referred to as basal or Malpighian.*

Blood and Lymph Supply to the Skin

From 1/2 to 2/3 of the total blood supply of the body is found distributed to the skin. The blood and lymph, as they circulate through the skin, contribute essential materials for growth, nourishment and repair of the skin, hair and nails. In the subcutaneous tissue are found networks of arteries and lymphatics which send their smaller branches to hair papillae, the hair follicles and the skin glands. The capillaries are quite numerous in the skin.

Nerves of the skin. The skin contains the surface endings of many nerve fibers classified as follows:

1. Motor nerve fibers, which are distributed to the blood vessels and the arrectores pili muscles attached to the hair follicles.

2. Sensory nerve fibers, which react to heat, cold, touch, pressure and pain.

3. Secretory nerve fibers, which are distributed to the sweat and oil glands of the skin.

Sensory Nerves of the Skin

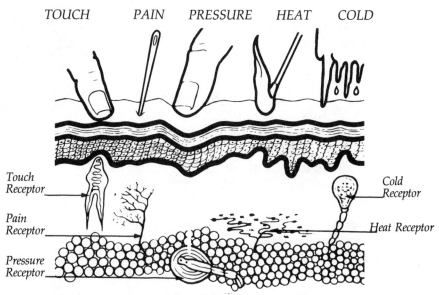

Sense of touch. The papillary layer of the dermis provides the body with the sense of touch. Nerves supplying the skin register basic types of sensations, namely: touch, pain, heat, cold, pressure, or deep touch. Nerve endings are most abundant in the fingertips. **Complex sensations,** such as vibrations, seem to depend on the sensitivity of a combination of these nerve endings.

Skin Elasticity

The **pliability of the skin** depends on the elasticity of the dermis. For example, healthy skin regains its former shape almost immediately after being expanded.

Aging skin. The aging process of the skin is a subject of vital importance to everyone. Perhaps the most outstanding characteristic of the aged skin is its loss of elasticity.

Skin Color

The **color of the skin,** whether fair, medium, or dark, depends in part on the blood supply to the skin, and primarily on the **melanin,** or coloring matter, that is deposited in the stratum germinativum and the papillary layers of the dermis. The pigment's color varies in different people. The distinctive color of the skin is a hereditary trait and varies among races and nationalities.

The Glands of the Skin

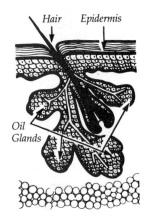

Hair   Epidermis

*Oil
Glands*

**BODY HAIR
AND FOLLICLE**
*Body hair (lanugo) with
multiple oil (sebaceous)
glands.*

The skin contains two types of duct glands that extract materials from the blood to form new substances.

1. The **sudoriferous** *(su-dor-if'er-us)*, or **sweat, glands** excrete sweat.

2. The **sebaceous** *(se-bay'shus)*, or **oil, glands** secrete sebum.

The **sweat glands** (tubular type) consist of a coiled base, or **fundus** *(fun'dus)*, and a tube-like duct which terminates at the skin surface to form the **sweat pore.** Practically all parts of the body are supplied with sweat glands, which are more numerous on the palms, soles, forehead, and in the armpits.

The sweat glands regulate body temperature and help to eliminate waste products from the body. Their activity is greatly increased by heat, exercise, emotions, and certain drugs.

The excretion of sweat is under the control of the nervous system. Normally, 1-2 pints (.47-.95 l) of liquids containing salts are eliminated daily through the sweat pores in the skin.

The **oil glands** (saccular type) consist of little sacs whose ducts open into the hair follicles. They secrete **sebum** *(se'bum)*, which lubricates the skin and preserves the softness of the hair. With the

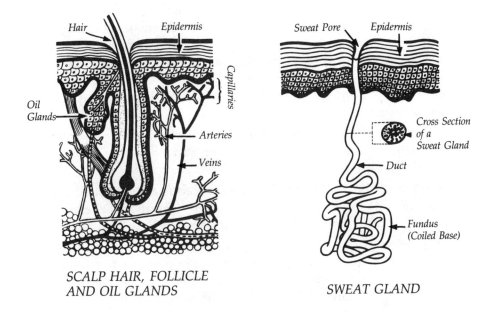

SCALP HAIR, FOLLICLE
AND OIL GLANDS

SWEAT GLAND

exception of the palms and soles, these glands are found in all parts of the body, particularly in the face.

Sebum is an oily substance produced by the oil glands. Ordinarily, it flows through the oil ducts leading to the mouths of the hair follicles. However, when the sebum becomes hardened and the duct becomes clogged, a **blackhead** is formed. Cleanliness is of prime importance in keeping the skin free of blemishes.

Functions of the Skin

The principal functions of the skin are protection, sensation, heat regulation, excretion, secretion, and absorption.

1. **Protection.** The skin protects the body from injury and bacterial invasion. The outermost layer of the epidermis is covered with a thin layer of sebum, thus rendering it waterproof. It is resistant to wide variations in temperature, minor injuries, chemically active substances, and many microbes.

2. **Sensation.** Through its sensory nerve endings, the skin responds to heat, cold, touch, pressure, and pain. Extreme stimulation of a sensory nerve ending produces pain. A minor burn is very painful, but a deep burn that destroys the nerves may be painless. Sensory endings, responsive to touch and pressure, are situated near hair follicles.

3. **Heat regulation.** The healthy body maintains a constant internal temperature of about 98.6° Fahrenheit (37° Celsius). As changes occur in the outside temperature, the blood and sweat glands of the skin make necessary adjustments in their functions. Heat regulation is a function of the skin, the organ that protects the body from the environment. The body is cooled by the evaporation of sweat.

4. **Excretion.** Perspiration from the sweat glands is excreted from the skin. Water lost by perspiration carries salt and other chemicals with it.

5. **Secretion.** Sebum is secreted by the sebaceous glands. Excessive flow of oil from the oil glands may produce **seborrhea** *(seb-o-ree′a)*. Emotional stress may increase the flow of sebum.

6. **Absorption** is limited, but it does occur. Cosmetic ingredients may enter the body through the skin and influence it to a minor degree. These ingredients must be of small enough molecular weight to penetrate the hair follicles and sebaceous gland openings.

The skin has an immunity to many things that touch it or gain entry into it.

Appendages of the skin are hair, nails, and sweat and oil glands.

THE SKIN: A Review

1. **Briefly describe the skin.**	The skin is a slightly moist, soft, strong, flexible covering of the body.
2. **What are five important functions of the skin?**	Protection, heat regulation, secretion and excretion, sensation, and absorption.
3. **Name the two main divisions of the skin.**	The epidermis and dermis.
4. **Briefly describe the structure of the epidermis.**	The epidermis forms the outer protective covering of the skin of the body, does not contain any blood vessels, but has many small nerve endings.
5. **Name the layers of the epidermis.**	1. Stratum corneum (horny layer). 2. Stratum lucidum (clear layer) 3. Stratum granulosum (granular layer). 4. Stratum mucosum (germinative, basal or Malpighian layer).
6. **Which epidermal layer is continually being shed and replaced?**	Stratum corneum.
7. **Which epidermal layer consists of small, transparent cells?**	Stratum lucidum.
8. **Which epidermal layer starts to undergo a change into a horny substance?**	Stratum granulosum.
9. **Where is the coloring matter of the skin found?**	In the deepest layer of the stratum mucosum of the epidermis and the papillary layer of the dermis.
10. **Which layer of the epidermis is responsible for its reproduction and growth?**	The deepest layer of the stratum mucosum which is sometimes called stratum germinativum.
11. **Describe the structure of the dermis.**	Consists of an elastic network of cells containing blood and lymph vessels, nerve endings, sweat glands, oil glands and hair follicles.
12. **Name the two layers of the dermis.**	The papillary layer and the reticular layer.

THE SKIN: A Review (continued)

13. Name two structures found in the papillary layer of the dermis.	Looped capillaries and tactile corpuscles.
14. Which structures are found in the reticular layers?	Fat cells, blood and lymph vessels, sweat and oil glands and hair follicles.
15. What renders the skin flexible?	The elastic fibers in the dermis.
16. List three important functions of the subcutaneous tissue.	Acts as a protective cushion for outer skin, gives smoothness and contour to the body and also contains fats for use as energy.
17. About how much blood is found in the skin?	From one-half to two-thirds of the total blood supply in the body is found in the skin.
18. Name three types of nerve fibers found in the skin.	Motor, sensory and secretory nerve fibers.
19. To what structures in the skin are the motor nerve fibers distributed?	They are distributed to blood vessels and muscles attached to hair follicles.
20. To what five things will the sensory nerves of the skin react?	They react to the sense of heat, cold, touch, pressure and pain.
21. What are the functions of the nerve fibers distributed to sweat and oil glands?	They regulate the excretion of perspiration from sweat glands and control the flow of sebum to the surface of the skin.
22. What regulates the temperature of the body?	The blood circulation through the skin and perspiration produced by the sweat glands.
23. What is the normal temperature of the human body?	98.6 degrees Fahrenheit.

SWEAT AND OIL GLANDS: A Review (continued)

1. **What is a gland?**	An organ which removes certain materials from the blood and forms new substances.
2. **Name two types of glands found in the skin.**	Sudoriferous or sweat glands; sebaceous or oil glands.
3. **Describe the structure of the sweat glands.**	Consist of a coiled base and a tube-like duct which forms a pore at the surface of the skin.
4. **Where are sweat glands found?**	Over the entire area of the skin, more numerous on the palms, soles, forehead and armpits.
5. **What is the function of the sweat glands?**	Help to eliminate waste products in the form of sweat.
6. **What four things will increase the activity of the sweat glands?**	Heat, exercise, mental excitement and certain drugs.
7. **Describe the structure of the oil glands.**	They consist of small sacs whose ducts open into the neck of the hair follicle.
8. **Which substance is secreted by the oil glands?**	Sebum, an oily substance.
9. **What is the chief function of sebum?**	Lubricates the skin and hair, keeping them soft and pliable.
10. **On what part of the body are oil glands found?**	Oil glands are found in all parts of the body with the exception of the palms and soles.

BONES

Bone is the hardest structure of the body. Its function is to give shape and strength to the body and to keep the various parts and organs in position.

Bones of the Arm and Hand

The **upper extremities** consist of the shoulders, arms, wrist and hands.

Shoulder. Each side of the shoulder is made up of one clavicle and one scapula, forming the back of the shoulder.

The **bones in the arm** are:

1. **Humerus** (hew'mer-us)—Longest and largest bone of the upper arm.

2. **Ulna** (ul'na)—The large bone on little finger side of forearm.

3. **Radius** (ray'de-us)—The small bone on thumb side of forearm.

The **carpus** (kar'pus) (the wrist)—A flexible joint composed of eight small, irregular bones, held together by ligaments.

The bones of the wrist are:

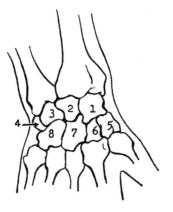

Bones of the Wrist

Upper row—start at thumb side.
1. Navicular (scaphoid)
2. Lunate (semilunar)
3. Triangular (cuneiform)
4. Pisiform.

Lower row—start at thumb side.
5. Greater multangular (trapezium)
6. Lesser multangular (trapezoid)
7. Capitate (Os magnum)
8. Hamate (Unciform)

Bones of the Arm and Hand
Anterior View—Palm Side of Hand

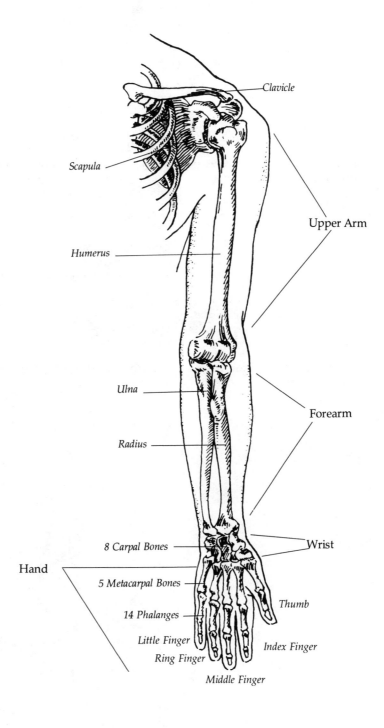

Clavicle

Scapula

Upper Arm

Humerus

Ulna

Forearm

Radius

8 Carpal Bones

Wrist

Hand

5 Metacarpal Bones

Thumb

14 Phalanges

Little Finger

Index Finger

Ring Finger

Middle Finger

The hand is divided into two regions:

1. The **metacarpus** *(met-a-kar'pus)* or **palm**—Consists of five long, slender bones, called the first, second, third, fourth, and fifth metacarpal bones, respectively.

2. The **digits** *(dij'its)*—Consist of three phalanges *(fa-lan'jeez)* or bones in each finger, and two in the thumb, totaling 14 bones.

The **names** of the **fingers** are the thumb, index or forefinger, middle, ring, and little or pinky.

BONES OF THE ARM AND HAND: A Review

1. Name the principal bones of the arm and hand.	Humerus, ulna, radius, carpus (wrist), metacarpus (palm), phalanges (digits).
2. Locate the arm bones.	Humerus—long bone of the upper arm. Ulna—large bone on little finger side of forearm. Radius—small bone on thumb side of the forearm.
3. How many bones are found in the wrist, palm and digits of the hand?	Wrist—8 bones. Palm—5 bones. Digits—14 bones.
4. What are the common names for the fingers of the hand?	Thumb, index or forefinger, middle, ring and little finger or pinky.

MUSCLES

Muscle is a contractile, elastic, fibrous tissue. Muscles cover, shape and support the skeleton, and their function is to produce all movements of the body. Muscles rely upon the skeleton and the nervous system for their activities.

Muscles are attached to bones, cartilage, ligaments, tendons, skin and somtimes to each other.

There are over 500 muscles, large and small, comprising approximately 40% to 50% of the weight of the body.

Muscles of the Arm and Hand

The principal muscles which attach the arms to the trunk and permit movements of the shoulders and arms are:

1. **Trapezius** *(tra-pee'zee-us)* and **latissimus dorsi** *(la-tis'i-mus dor'sy)* — Cover the upper and middle region of the back.

2. **Pectoralis** *(pek-tor-al'is)* **major** and **pectoralis minor** — Cover the front of the chest.

The principal muscles of the upper arm and shoulder are:

1. **Deltoid** *(del'toyd)* — The Large, thick, triangular-shaped muscle shapes the shoulder, lifts and turns the arm.

2. **Biceps** *(by'seps)* (biceps brachii) — The two-headed and principal muscle on the front of the upper arm. It lifts the forearm, flexes the elbow, and turns the palm downward.

3. **Triceps** *(try'seps)* (triceps brachii) — The three-headed muscle of the arm, which covers the entire back of the upper arm, and extends the forearm forward.

Muscles of the Forearm

The forearm is made up of a series of muscles and strong tendons. The manicurist is concerned with the following:

1. **Pronators** *(pro-nay'tors)* — The most important of the group; turn the hand inward, so that the palm faces downward.

2. **Supinators** *(sew-pinay'tors)* — Turn the hand outward, and the palm upward.

3. **Flexors** *(flek'sors)* — Bend the wrist, and draw the hand and close fingers toward the forearm.

4. **Extensors** *(eks-ten'sors)* — Straighten the wrist, hand and fingers to form a straight line.

Muscles of the Arm and Hand

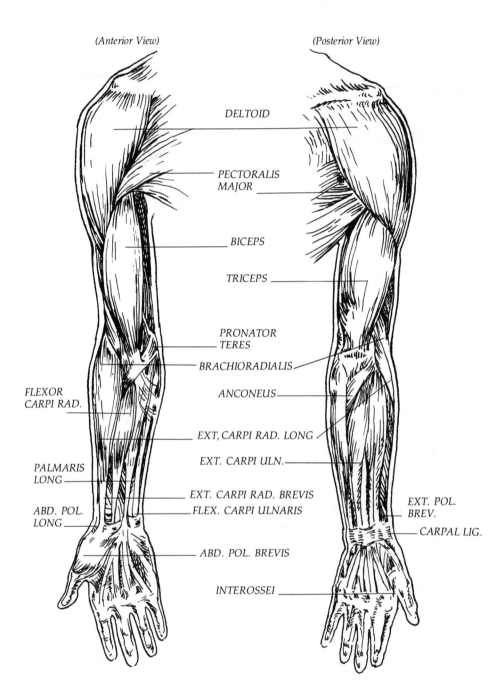

(Anterior View)   *(Posterior View)*

DELTOID

PECTORALIS
MAJOR

BICEPS

TRICEPS

PRONATOR
TERES

BRACHIORADIALIS

FLEXOR
CARPI RAD.

ANCONEUS

EXT. CARPI RAD. LONG

EXT. CARPI ULN.

PALMARIS
LONG

ABD. POL.
LONG

EXT. CARPI RAD. BREVIS
FLEX. CARPI ULNARIS

EXT. POL.
BREV.

CARPAL LIG.

ABD. POL. BREVIS

INTEROSSEI

Muscles of the Hand

The hand has many small muscles overlapping from joint to joint, imparting flexibility and strength. When the hands are properly cared for, these muscles will remain supple and graceful. They close and open the hands and fingers.

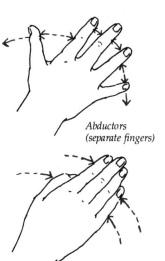

Abductors
(separate fingers)

Adductors
(draw fingers together)

Abductor *(ab-duk'tor)* and **adductor** *(a-duk'tor)* muscles—located in the thumb and fingers, at the base of the digits. The abductor muscles separate the fingers and the adductor muscles draw them together.

MUSCLES OF THE ARM AND HAND: A Review

1. **What are the principal muscles of the upper arm and shoulder?**	Deltoid, biceps and triceps.
2. **Name four types of muscles which control the movement of the forearms.**	Pronators, supinators, flexors and extensors.
3. **Distinguish between the functions of the pronator and supinator muscles.**	The pronators turn the palm downward. The supinators turn the palm upward.
4. **Distinguish between the flexor and extensor muscles.**	The flexor muscles bend the wrist and fingers. The extensor muscles straighten out the hand and fingers.
5. **Distinguish between the functions of the abductor and adductor muscles.**	The abductor muscles separate the fingers. The adductor muscles draw the fingers together.

NERVES

Nerves control and coordinate the functions of all the other parts of the body and makes them work harmoniously and efficiently.

The **functions** of nerves are:

1. To rule the body by controlling all visible and invisible activities.

2. To control human thoughts and conduct.

3. To govern all internal and external movements of the body.

4. To give the power to see, hear, move, talk, feel, think and remember.

A **neuron** *(new'ron)* is the structural unit of the nervous system. It is composed of a nerve cell and its outgrowth of long and short fibers, called **cell processes.** The nerve cell stores energy and nutriment for the cell processes which convey the nerve impulses throughout the body. Practically all the nerve cells are contained in the brain and spinal cord.

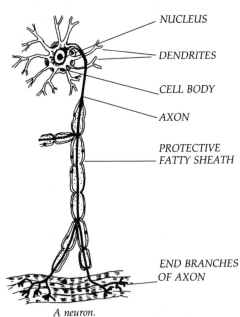

NUCLEUS

DENDRITES

CELL BODY

AXON

PROTECTIVE
FATTY SHEATH

END BRANCHES
OF AXON

A neuron.

Nerves are long white cords made up of fibers (cell processes) from nerve cells. They have their origin in the brain and spinal cord, and distribute branches to all parts of the body. Nerves furnish both sensation and motion.

Types of Nerves

Sensory nerves, termed **afferent** *(af'er-ent)* **nerves,** carry impulses or messages from sense organs to the brain, where sensations of touch, cold, heat, sight, hearing, taste and pain are experienced.

Motor nerves, termed **efferent nerves,** carry impulses from the brain to the muscles, the transmitted impulses causing movement.

Nerves of the Arm and Hand

The principal nerves supplying the superficial parts of the arm and hand are:

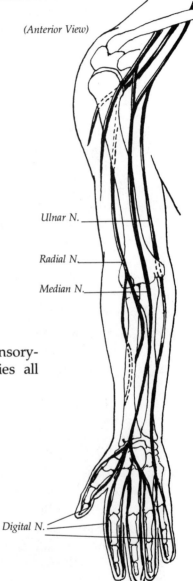

(Anterior View)

1. **The ulnar** *(ul'nar)* **nerve** (sensory-motor)—With its branches, supplies the little finger side of the arm, and the palm of the hand.

2. **The radial** *(ray'dee-al)* **nerve** (sensory-motor)—With its branches, supplies the thumb side of the arm and the back of the hand.

Ulnar N.

Radial N.

Median N.

3. **The median** *(mee'dee'an)* **nerve** (sensory-motor)—A smaller nerve than the ulnar and radial nerves. With its branches, supplies the arm and hand.

4. **The digital** *(dij'i-tal)* **nerves**—(sensory-motor)—With its branches, supplies all fingers of the hand.

Digital N.

NERVES OF THE ARM AND HAND: A Review

1. Name and locate the principal nerves of the arms and hands.	The ulnar nerve supplies the little finger side of the arm and palm of the hand. The radial nerve supplies the thumb side of the arm and back of the hand.

BLOOD CIRCULATION

Blood is circulated through the body in a steady stream, by means of the heart and blood vessels, whose functions it is to supply body cells with nourishment and carry away waste products.

The Blood Vessels

The arteries, capillaries and veins transport blood to and from the heart and the various tissues of the body. The main artery of the body is the **aorta**, which starts from the left ventricle of the heart and subdivides into smaller arteries.

Arteries *(ar'ter-eez)* are thick-walled muscular and elastic vessels that carry pure blood from the heart to the capillaries. They vary in size from the aorta, which is about an inch (2.5 cm) in diameter, to others which are a small fraction of an inch.

Capillaries *(kap'i-ler-eez)* are minute, thin-walled blood vessels whose network is to connect the smaller arteries with the veins. Through their walls, the tissues receive nourishment and eliminate waste products.

Veins *(vainz)* are thin-walled blood vessels containing cup-like valves to prevent backflow, and carrying impure blood from the various parts of the body back to the heart.

Blood Supply of the Arm and Hand

The **ulnar** *(ul'nar)* and **radial** *(ray'dee-al)* **arteries** are the main blood vessels for the arm and hand. They branch from the brachial artery and extend down the inner and outer sides of the arm. The ulnar artery and its numerous branches supply the little finger side of the arm and the palm of the hand. The radial artery and its branches supply the thumb side of the arm and the back of the hand.

Veins. The important veins are almost parallel to the arteries and have the same names as the arteries. Whereas the arteries are found deeper in the tissues, the veins lie nearer to the surface of the arms and hands.

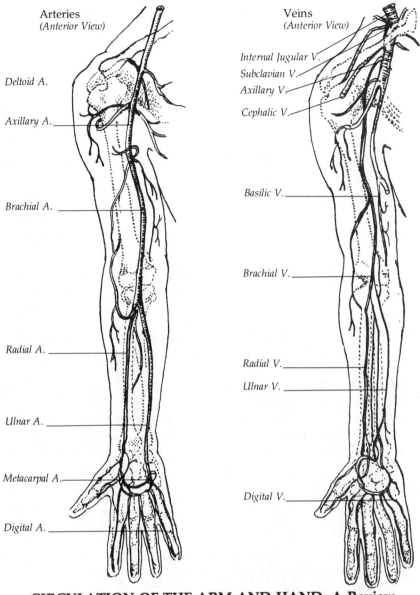

Arteries
(Anterior View)

Deltoid A.

Axillary A.

Brachial A.

Radial A.

Ulnar A.

Metacarpal A.

Digital A.

Veins
(Anterior View)

Internal Jugular V.
Subclavian V.
Axillary V.
Cephalic V.

Basilic V.

Brachial V.

Radial V.
Ulnar V.

Digital V.

CIRCULATION OF THE ARM AND HAND: A Review

1. Name the principal blood vessels of the arm and hand.	The ulnar and radial arteries and the ulnar and radial veins.
2. Which artery supplies the little finger side of the arm and palm of the hand?	The ulnar artery.
3. Which artery supplies the thumb side of the arm?	The radial artery.

FIRST AID

Emergencies arise in every line of business, and a knowledge of first aid measures is invaluable to the salon manager and staff.

A physician (or emergency ambulance) should be called as soon as possible after any accident has occurred, both as a courtesy to the client and as a protection to the salon. There are certain first aid treatments, however, that the layman can give while awaiting medical assistance. Have a well equipped first aid kit where it is within easy access. When possible the salon owner, manager, and employees should take a course in first aid.

For more information about emergency care, consult the latest edition of the First Aid Manual published by the American Red Cross.

Abrasions. When the skin is cut or broken by accident, the skin should be gently closed and an antiseptic should be applied.

Burns. Burns may be caused by electricity or flames, while scalds usually are due to exposure to hot liquids or live steam. Burns are classified as first degree, characterized by redness; second degree, having watery blisters; and third degree, involving deeper structures of the flesh with possible charring of tissues. In case of accidental burns, see that the client gets immediate medical attention by a physician.

A quick, safe, and temporarily effective method of treating burns is to immediately apply cold water to the affected area.

Electric shock. The clothing should be loosened and the client removed to a cool place. The head should be raised and the tongue drawn forward to prevent strangulation. Apply artificial respiration. Stimulants should not be given.

Heat exhaustion. Heat exhaustion is a general functional depression due to heat. It is characterized by a cool, moist skin and collapse. Clothing should be loosened and the client removed to a cool, dark, quiet place. The client should be kept lying down for several hours, as rest and quiet will hasten recovery.

Nosebleed. Nosebleed is a hemorrhage from the nose, and is treated by loosening the collar and applying pads saturated with cool water to the face and back of the neck.

Foreign body in the eye. If this is under the lower lid, pull the lid down gently while the client looks up. If the hair or speck of dust can be seen, it should be removed with the corner of a clean, moistened handkerchief or with a twist of clean cotton.

If it is under the upper lid, pull the lid down over the eye and the speck should then be apparent when the client opens his or her eye again. Remove in same way as above.

Fainting. Fainting is caused by a lack of blood flow to the brain, bad air, indigestion, nervous condition, unpleasant odors, etc., and is characterized by pallor and loss of muscular control. There is a temporary suspension of respiration and circulation. If there is a sign of fainting and before it actually occurs have the client hold his/her head between the knees, as this action may check the faintness by causing the blood to flow quickly to the head. **Treatment for fainting** consists of loosening all tight clothing, being sure there is fresh air in the room, and placing the client in a reclining position with the head slightly lower than the body. If the client is conscious, hold aromatic spirits of ammonia near his/her nose or offer stimulants, such as hot coffee, tea, or milk. If the client is unconscious, apply cold applications to the face, chest, and over the heart. Do not dash cold water in the client's face.

Epileptic seizure. An epileptic fit is a nerve disorder characterized by unconsciousness, convulsions, contortions of the face, foaming at the mouth, and rolling of the eyes. In such a case, call for immediate medical attention.

Emergency treatment consists of lying client on the side and fixing a wad of cotton between the teeth to prevent biting of the tongue. Mild stimulants may be administered in moderation after recovery. If the client falls into a deep sleep after the attack, he/she should not be disturbed, but allowed to awaken naturally.

In case of emergency. Every salon should have information that may be needed in case of an emergency, posted or placed (in clear view) near the telephone. The owner of the salon or manager should have the names, addresses, and telephone numbers of employees on file in case of an emergency. The file that is kept for regular clients also should have information that might be needed in case of an emergency. Addresses and telephone numbers for the following services should be placed near the salon telephone: fire station; police (local and state); emergency ambulance; nearest hospital emergency room; doctors; taxi service; telephone company and telephone numbers of persons and organizations that provide service.

Utility service companies, such as electricity, water, heat, air-conditioning, etc. also should be posted. Additional information to be included are the names and telephone numbers of the owner and/or manager, custodian, and others who might need to be called if something goes wrong in the salon.

Each employee should know where exits are located and how to evacuate a building quickly in case of fire or other emergencies. Fire extinguishers should be placed where they can be reached easily, and employees should know how to use them. A well-stocked first aid kit should be kept within easy reach.

Artificial Respiration

To deal with occurrences such as severe electric shock, protracted fainting, poisoning, and gas suffocation, the most currently acceptable methods are mouth-to-mouth breathing or mouth-to-nose breathing.

Procedure

1. Place client on a flat surface.

2. Place one hand on back of client's neck, one hand on forehead, and tilt the head backward until the chin is pointed upward.

3. Lift client's lower jaw forward to move the tongue away from the throat.

4. Pinch client's nose closed.

5. Seal your mouth on client's mouth and give four quick breaths.

6. Listen for client's breathing and check pulse. (Pulse can be checked by placing fingers on carotid artery.)

7. If there is no pulse, continue giving at least one breath every five seconds until you see client's chest rising and falling.

8. For mouth-to-nose breathing, follow the same procedure as for mouth-to-mouth breathing, except that you close the client's mouth with your hand and blow into the nose.

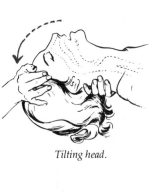

Tilting head.

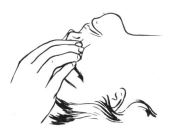

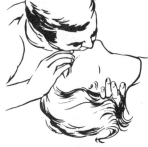

Giving four quick breaths.

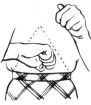

Checking pulse.

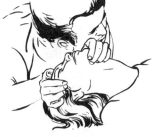

Checking breathing.

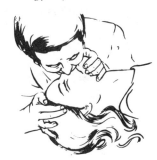

Mouth-to-nose breathing

Procedure for Breathing Obstruction (Abdominal Thrust)

If the client's breathing becomes obstructed due to choking, immediate help must be given.

Procedure

1. Standing behind client, hit rapidly between the shoulder blades.
2. Wrap your arms around client's waist. Make a fist and place the thumb just below the breastbone.
3. Hold your fist with your other hand and press it into client's abdomen, using four quick upward thrusts.
4. Repeat the procedure if necessary.

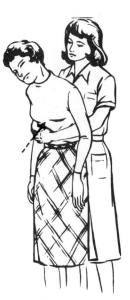

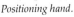

Positioning hand.

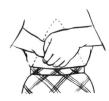

Positioning hand.

Thrusting upward.

FIRST AID: A Review

1. When an accident occurs, when should a physician be called?	As soon as possible.
2. What should be done when the skin is accidentally cut?	An antiseptic should be applied.
3. What causes heat exhaustion?	A general functional depression due to heat
4. How is a nosebleed treated?	By loosening the collar and applying pads saturated with cool water to the face and back of the neck.
5. Give the procedure for the abdominal thrust.	Stand behind client. Hit client rapidly between the shoulder blades. Wrap your arms around client's waist. Make a fist and place the thumb just below the breastbone. Hold your fist with your other hand and press it into client's abdomen, using four quick upward thrusts. Repeat procedure if necessary.

Success in the Salon

Nail care is rapidly advancing as a popular segment of the field of cosmetology. To take full advantage of the growing interest in manicuring, the manicurist must develop professionalism and good business sense.

Whether you open your own salon or work in someone else's, how you handle yourself during working hours will determine whether or not you're a professional and a financial success.

BOOKING APPOINTMENTS

Booking appointments must be done with care, because the efficient scheduling of appointments can make the difference between success and failure. Services are sold in terms of time on the appointment page. Depending on how it is used, time may spell either a gain or a loss.

The size of the salon determines who books the appointments. This may be done by a full-time receptionist, the owner or manager, or any of the stylists or manicurists working in the salon.

GOOD BUSINESS ADMINISTRATION

Good business administration requires the keeping of a simple and efficient record system. Records are of value only if they are correct, concise, and complete. Bookkeeping means keeping an accurate record of all income and expenses. Income is usually classified as receipts from services and retail sales. Expenses include rent, utilities, insurance, salaries, advertising, equipment, and repairs. The assistance of an accountant is recommended to help keep records accurate. Retain check stubs, cancelled checks, receipts, and invoices.

Proper business records are necessary to meet the requirements of local, state, and federal laws regarding taxes and employees.

All business transactions must be recorded in order to maintain proper records. These are required by the owner, or manager, for the following reasons:

1. For efficient operation of the salon.

2. For determining income, expenses, profit or loss.

3. For proving the value of the salon to prospective buyers.

4. For arranging a bank loan.

5. For such reports as income tax, social security, unemployment and disability insurance, wage and hour law, accident, compensation and labor tax.

Daily Records

Keeping daily records enables the owner, or manager, to know just how the business is progressing. A weekly or monthly summary helps to:

1. Make comparisons with other years.
2. Detect any changes in demands for different services.
3. Order necessary supplies.
4. Check on the use of materials according to the type of service rendered.
5. Control expenses and waste.

Each expense item affects the total gross income. Accurate records show the cost of operation in relation to income.

Keep daily sales slips, appointment book, and a petty cash book for at least six months. Payroll book, cancelled checks, monthly and yearly records are usually held for at least seven years. Service and inventory records also are important to keep. Sales records help to maintain a perpetual inventory which can be used to:

1. Prevent overstocking.
2. Prevent running short of supplies needed for services.
3. Help in establishing the net worth of the business at the end of the year.

Service Records

A service record should be kept of treatments given and merchandise sold to each client. Such information is the basis for suggested services that result in increased sales. For this purpose, use a card file system or memorandum book.

All service records should contain the name and address of the client, date, amount charged, product used, and results obtained. Also, note the client's preferences and taste.

Keep a running inventory of all supplies. Classify them as to their use and retail value. Those to be used in the business are **consumption** supplies. Those to be sold are **retail** supplies.

Inventory records indicate which merchandise is most popular, and prevent running short of any item. When reordering, buy enough merchandise that can be used or sold within a reasonable period of time. It is better to have a slight excess rather than a deficiency of supplies.

Appointment Record

The use of a private appointment record helps the manicurist arrange working time to suit the client's convenience. The appointment book accurately reflects what is taking place in the salon at a given time. The manicurist who makes advance preparation can render prompt and efficient service when the client arrives. Waste in time and money is prevented.

Answering Price Objections

A client may ask for the price of a nail wrap. After being told what the cost is, the client says, "I can get the same nail wrap around the corner for less." How will you answer this objection?

The best way to overcome such an objection is to build up more value in the client's mind. You can appeal to his or her better judgment by presenting logical reasons. Try to show the client how he or she will profit from the greater value and better service offered by your beauty salon.

In the conversation, first get the client to agree with you. You might say in a calm, assuring voice, "I quite agree, Mrs. Brown, but you can also get a pair of shoes for less. Yet, you prefer to pay more and get only the best for your feet. Why, Mrs. Brown? Because you know that although shoes may look the same, there may be a vast difference in the quality of the leather, the skill of the shoemaker, and the fit of the shoes. In the long run, the higher-priced shoe will give you better wear, and, therefore, cost less.

"By the same token, our nail wrap costs more because we use only the highest quality materials for your nails, and take great care to produce natural-looking nails. You can rest assured that the reason we charge more is to enable us to provide you with better service and a higher quality nail wrap."

PROPER TELEPHONE USAGE

1. Be prompt. When the telephone rings, answer it immediately, after the first ring, if possible.
2. Be prepared. Know in advance what you intend to say. Be able to provide accurate information to any inquirer. Always keep a pencil, ball point pen and pad handy for messages.

3. Identify both yourself and your salon for every incoming and outgoing call.

4. Speak clearly into the phone. Don't mumble or shout. Use good English and avoid slang.

5. Be tactful and courteous when speaking over the phone. Refer to the caller by last name. Try to leave a good impression on your listener.

6. Be interested in and helpful to the people who call the beauty salon.

7. Avoid arguments and interruptions while on the phone.

SELLING IN THE BEAUTY SALON

Selling is becoming an increasingly important responsibility of the manicurist. The manicurist who is equally proficient as both a nail technician and a salesperson is most likely to be the one to succeed in business.

No attempt is made here to cover all aspects of selling, but if students use this material as a basis upon which to build, they will find that effective selling techniques will become part of their repertoire of skills.

Successful salesmanship requires ambition and determination. Effective salesmanship is a necessity in any business.

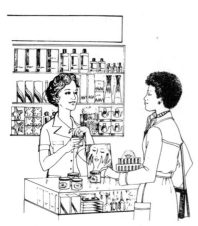

The first step in selling is to "sell yourself." Clients must like and trust the manicurist in order for them to buy beauty services or merchandise.

Every client who enters a salon is a prospective purchaser of additional services or merchandise. The manner in which you greet him or her lays the foundation for suggestive selling. Greet the client with a smile and say, "May I help you?" Be ready and eager to serve clients. Recognizing the needs and preferences of clients makes the intelligent use of suggestive selling possible.

Selling Principles

The manicurist who is to become a proficient salesperson must understand, and be able to apply, the following principles of selling:

1. Be familiar with the merits and benefits of each service and product.
2. Adapt the approach and selling method to the needs and psychology of each client.
3. Be self-confident. It is essential to make selling agreeable and productive.
4. Stimulate attention, interest, and desire, all of which lead up to a sale.
5. Never misrepresent your service or product.
6. Use tact in handling a client. Avoid being rude or offensive.
7. Understand human nature so that you can apply appropriate sales techniques.
8. Don't be negative.
9. To sell a product or service, deliver a sales talk in a relaxed, friendly manner and, if possible, demonstrate its use.
10. Recognize the right psychological moment to close any sale.

Types of Clients and Ways of Handling Them

The manicurist who is most likely to be successful in selling additional services or merchandise to clients is the one who can recognize the many different types of people and knows how to handle each type.

The following material describes seven of the most common types you are likely to deal with, and suggests ways on how each should be treated.

1. **Shy, timid types.** Make them feel at ease. Lead the conversation. Don't force them to talk. Cheer them up.
2. **Talkative types.** Be a good, patient listener. Tactfully switch the conversation to their beauty needs.
3. **Nervous, irritable types.** These people do not want much conversation. They want a fast worker and efficient service. Get them started and finished as fast as possible.

4. **Inquisitive, over-cautious types.** Explain everything in detail. Show them facts—sealed bottled, brand names. Ask their opinion.

5. **Conceited "know-it-all" types.** Agree with them. Cater to their vanity. Suggest things in question form. Don't argue with them. Compliment them.

6. **Teenagers.** Don't oversell them. Give them special advice on nail care and proper products.

7. **The elderly** (60 and over). Be exra courteous and solicitious of their comfort. Suggest a nail length and polish becoming to a mature person.

Personality in Selling

Greeting the client. Your selling power will increase progressively as you make clients aware of your personal interst in their welfare. Treat clients with friendliness and extend such little courtesies as a warm greeting and a pleasant smile. Hang up client's coat in designated area, and do not let him or her wait too long for service. Attention to these little details is greatly appreciated by clients. The beauty service may be obtained elsewhere, but the personality and friendliness behind the service are what bring the client back again to you.

Personal magnetism is a valuable asset in selling. Each person creates an atmosphere that may either attract or repel clients. Since an attractive personality is conducive to making friends and increasing sales, the manicurist should develop the qualities that make for an outstanding personality.

The following are positive qualities necessary for a successful selling career:

Optimism—the expectation that things will come out all right.

Acquisitiveness—the desire to acquire wealth and improve one's position in life.

Self-assertiveness—the ability to face and overcome problems and obstacles.

Initiative—the ability to do what is necessary without being told what or how to do it.

Cheerfulness—a congenial spirit that makes the work of selling agreeable both the manicurist and the client.

Tact—saying or doing the right thing, at the right time, in the right place, without offense.

Sincerity—making your suggestions because you really believe the sale will be a good one for the client.

Ability to smile—a smiling face tells the client that you are pleased to be of service to him or her.

SALES PSYCHOLOGY

No matter how good a beauty service or product may be, you will find it difficult to make a sale if there is no need for it. Every person who enters a salon is an individual with specific wants and needs. Determine how the client can use a particular item before attempting to sell it.

Motives for buying. What are the motives that prompt people to buy beauty services and merchandise? People want to make the most of their natural endowments or substitute for what is lacking. Personal influence and social prestige can be enhanced by a youthful appearance. Vanity, personal satisfaction, and esthetic gratification are other reasons why clients desire beauty services. The buying motive that predominates and is the strongest is the one to which the manicurist should make his or her most successful appeal.

Help client make decision. If a client is doubtful or undecided, help him or her make a decision by giving honest and sincere advice. For instance, if a client wants sculptured nails and you see that her nails have a fungus condition, it is your responsibility to recommend that a physician be consulted first.

In the beauty profession, you should instill ideas in conjunction with selling services and merchandise. Show the client not only what the beauty service is, but also what it can mean to him or her in terms of results and benefits. Sell the idea that a beauty treatment or product will improve attractiveness and personality. The selling of ideas along with beauty services gives greater value to the client and more sales to the manicurist.

Sales Technique

The best interests of the client should be your first consideration. Under no circumstances should you approach a client with the thought of the amount of money you can get. Sincerity and honesty are the foundation of good salesmanship.

Careful consideration on your part will acquaint you with the client's needs, and those needs can be fulfilled to the complete satisfaction of the client and to your financial advantage. Tact and diplomacy must be used, as well as courtesy.

Use Attractive Displays

To acquaint new and regular clients with the quality and cost of beauty services and merchandise, use attractive displays in the window, at the reception desk, cosmetic counter, service booth, and boutique area. Dress the windows so that they carry a definite message and appeal to the people passing the salon. Frequent rearrangement of case displays and changes in the featured service or merchandise will draw attention to new items. Price signs should accompany the placards. If the price is within reach of the client, there will be no hesitation or embarrassment in obtaining more particulars about the advertisement.

An effective display can create interest in a particular service or product and help in its sale. Beauty products should appeal to the eye through color and to the imagination through suggestion of increased attractiveness. Manufacturers and wholesale dealers will cooperate in arranging for well-lighted and attractive displays of their products.

Describe Benefits of Beauty Service

Each nail service requires a suitable sales technique, employing simple and suggestive language that will make the client feel like buying. In creating interest and desire, use picture words and descriptive adjectives charged with feeling. Present to the client a verbal picture of that person as a relaxed, refreshed, and more charming individual after using the recommended service.

Nail sculpturing. Say to Mrs. Smith, "The sculptured nail procedure we use will give you long, luxurious nails that will look very natural. Your sculptured nails will prompt others to remark, 'What beautiful nails you have!'" An emotional appeal is often more effective than the use of cold, reasoned facts.

For salesmanship to be successful, the language should be positive rather than negative. Refrain from using the word "don't" in selling language.

Nail wrapping. A client makes an appointment for a basic manicure. Her nails are weak and short due to breaking and splitting. The conversation might be as follows:

Manicurist: "Mrs. Jones, your nails are a little weak. I'd like to do a silk wrap to make them stronger and to protect them while they grow. The silk wrap will help your nails become stronger and more uniform as they get longer."

Client: "I guess my nails are in poor condition. Please go ahead and do the silk wrap. I'd certainly like my nails to look more attractive."

Don't Underestimate Client

At no time should you underestimate either the client's intelligence or ability to pay for what he or she actually wants or needs. Simple attire and lack of pretentiousness on the part of the client are no indications that he or she is not able to afford anything he or she wants. Regardless of financial status, each client is entitled to courteous treatment and sincere consideration, whether the purchase is for a large or small amount. When making a sale, you should refrain from mentioning price until the client's interest is sufficiently aroused. Then it should be given in a casual manner, without attaching too much importance to it.

Selling Beauty Services and Accessories

Learn to identify clients not only by appearance, but also by name. Address the client as "Miss Jones" or "Mr. Smith" and not by "dearie" or "honey." Keep a reminder file of the client's special characteristics and problems, and the type and price of service rendered and merchandise sold. When the client calls again, you can refresh your memory as to previous work. Reminder forms help not only to sell more beauty services and products, but also assure the client that you have a personal interest in his or her problems.

Another source of income is keeping up with the latest nail care techniques and products.

In selling beauty services and merchandise, stress quality and other advantages over cheaper substitutes. The manicurist should have a ready answer for a price objection. She can say, "Although you are paying a higher price, you will be getting greater value and superior results from the money expended." The manicurist also can explain that the higher price is occasioned by the use of standard top quality materials and highly skilled manicurists.

Selling Supplies

Before the manicurist tries to sell accessory supplies, such as polish, creams, perfumes, atomizers, and jewelry, he or she should have correct information concerning the following:

1. Location of the product.
2. Name and brand of product.
3. Contents and price of product.
4. Comparative merits of similar products that differ in price.

There should be a complete assortment of beauty accessories to meet the demand and to fit the pocketbook of all clients. The range in shade and color should be large enough to suit everyone. The sale of one item leads to the sale of other items, if they are in stock. Reorder regularly, to assure a fresh and complete stock at all times.

Once the client begins to buy through the salon, he or she will establish the buying habit that will continue as long as high quality merchandise is sold.

SUCCESS IN THE SALON: A Review

1. **Why should booking appointments be done with care?**	Because the efficient scheduling of appointments can make the difference between success and failure.
2. **List five reasons why all business transactions should be recorded.**	For efficient operation of the salon; for determining income; expense, profit or loss; for proving the value of the salon to prospective buyers; for arranging a bank loan; for reports such as income tax, social security, unemployment and disability insurance, wage and hour law, accident, compensation and labor tax.
3. **List five things a daily record will help you to do.**	Make comparisons with other years; detect any changes in service demands; order necessary supplies; check on the use of materials according to the type of service rendered; control expenses and waste.
4. **What should a service record contain?**	Name and address of client; date, amount charged, product used; results obtained; and client's preferences and taste.
5. **Why should a manicurist keep an appointment record?**	To help arrange working time to suit the client's convenience.
6. **Give seven rules for proper telephone usage.**	Be prompt; be prepared; identify yourself and your salon for each call; speak clearly; be tactful and courteous; be interested and helpful; avoid arguments and interruptions.
7. **List the ten principles of selling.**	Be familiar with features and benefits of service or product. Adapt approach and selling method to the needs and psychology of each client. Be self-confident and agreeable. Stimulate attention, interest and desire. Never misrepresent service or product. Use tact; avoid being rude or offensive. Apply appropriate sales technique. Don't be negative.

	Deliver sales talk in a relaxed, friendly manner. Recognize the right psychological moment to close the sale.
8. **How should you handle a shy, timid client?**	Make them feel at ease. Lead the conversation. Don't force them to talk. Cheer them up.
9. **What is one of the most effective selling tools?**	Showing an actual treatment or application to clients.
10. **In what four areas must the manicurist have the correct information before trying to sell beauty accessories?**	Location of product. Name and brand of product. Contents and price of product. Comparitive features of similar products that differ in price.

METRIC SYSTEM

Wherever possible, metric equivalents are indicated in the text alongside the measurement system commonly used in the United States. Conversions have been made strictly in accordance with conversion tables and information supplied by the U.S. Department of Commerce.

Everyday Metric-Aid

Spoonfuls

¼ tsp. .... 1.25 milliliters
½ tsp. .... 2.5 milliliters
¾ tsp. .... 3.75 milliliters
1 tsp. .... 5 milliliters
¼ tbls. .... 3.75 milliliters
½ tbls. .... 7.5 milliliters
¾ tbls. .... 11.25 milliliters
1 tbls. .... 15 milliliters

Fluid Ounces

¼ oz. .... 7.5 milliliters
½ oz. .... 15 milliliters
¾ oz. .... 22.5 milliliters
1 oz. .... 30 milliliters

Cups

¼ cup .... 59 milliliters
⅓ cup .... 78 milliliters
½ cup .... 118 milliliters
⅔ cup .... 157 milliliters
¾ cup .... 177 milliliters
1 cup .... 236 milliliters

Pints-Quarts-Gallons

½ pint .... 236 milliliters
1 pint .... 473 milliliters
1 quart .... 946.3 milliliters
1 gallon .... 3785 milliliters

Weight in Ounces

¼ oz. .... 7.1 grams
½ oz. ....14.17 grams
¾ oz. .... 21.27 grams
1 oz. .... 28.35 grams

Pounds

¼ lb. .... .113 kilograms
½ lb. .... .227 kilograms
¾ lb. .... .340 kilograms
1 lb. .... .454 kilograms
2.205 lbs. .... 1 kilogram

Length

1 inch .... 2.544 centimeters
1 foot .... 30.48 centimeters
1 yard .... 91.44 centimeters
100 ft. .... 30.48 meters
1 mile .... 1.609 kilometers
50 mph ...... 80.45 kilometers/hr.

Temperature

32° F. .... 0° Celsius
68° F. .... 20° Celsius
212° F. .... 100° Celsius

Square Measure

1 sq. in. .... 6.452 sq. cm.
1 sq. ft. .... 929 sq. cm.
1 sq. yd. .... .8361 sq. meters
1 acre .... 4047 sq. meters

Volume

1 cup ⟶ 250 milliliters
200 milliliters
¾ cup ⟶ 150 milliliters
½ cup ⟶ 100 milliliters
¼ cup ⟶ 50 milliliters

5 milliliters = 1 teaspoon
15 milliliters = 1 tablespoon

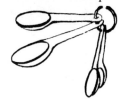

METRIC CONVERSION FACTORS

Approximate Conversions to Metric Measures

Symbol	When You Know	Multiply by	To Find	Symbol
Length (speed)				
in	inches	2.5	centimeters	cm
ft	feet	30	centimeters	cm
yd	yards	0.9	meters	m
mi	miles	1.6	kilometers	km
Area				
in²	square inches	6.5	square centimeters	cm²
ft²	square feet	0.09	square meters	m²
yd²	square yards	0.8	square meters	m²
mi²	square miles	2.6	square kilometers	km²
a	acres	0.4	hectares	ha
Mass (weight)				
oz	ounces	28	grams	g
lb	pounds	0.45	kilograms	kg
	short tons (2000 lb)	0.9	tonnes	t
Volume				
tsp	teaspoon	5	milliliters	ml
tbsp	tablespoon	15	milliliters	ml
fl oz	fluid ounces	30	milliliters	ml
c	cups	0.24	liters	l
pt	pints	0.47	liters	l
qt	quarts	0.95	liters	l
gal	gallons	3.8	liters	l
ft³	cubic feet	0.03	cubic meters	m³
yd³	cubic yards	0.76	cubic meters	m³
Temperature (exact)				
°F	Fahrenheit temperature	5/9 after subtracting 32)	Celsius temperature	°C

State Board Preparation
STATE BOARD EXAM REVIEW

1. The cuticle is composed of layers of the cells of the:
   1) epidermis
   3) matrix
   2) mantle
   4) dermis
   _____

2. Nails of adults grow at an average of:
   1) one-eighth of an inch a week
   3) one-twentieth of an inch a week
   2) one-eighth of an inch a month
   4) one-sixteenth of an inch a month
   _____

3. The matrix is well supplied with blood vessels and:
   1) lunula
   3) hyponychium
   2) nerves
   4) sebum
   _____

4. The technical term for the nail is:
   1) hyponychium
   3) eponychium
   2) onyx
   4) matrix
   _____

5. All growth of the nail takes place from its:
   1) eponychium
   3) cuticle
   2) groove
   4) matrix
   _____

6. Nails tend to grow faster:
   1) in winter
   3) in children
   2) in elderly people
   4) in fall
   _____

7. The part of the nail that extends over the fingertips is called the:
   1) free edge
   3) nail root
   2) matrix
   4) nail bed
   _____

8. The lunula is the visible half-moon at the:
   1) free edge of the nail
   3) base of the nail
   2) side of the nail
   4) groove of the nail
   _____

9. Nerves, blood and lymph vessels are found in the nail:
   1) plate
   3) lunula
   2) matrix
   4) keratin
   _____

10. The extension of excess cuticle at the base of the nail is known as the:
    1) hyponychium
    3) eponychium
    2) mantle
    4) perionychium
    _____

11. The deep fold of skin in which the nail root is lodged is called the:
    1) mantle
    3) eponychium
    2) nail groove
    4) lunula
    _____

12. The nail grooves are furrowed edges at the:
    1) base of the nail   3) root of the nail
    2) sides of the nail   4) free edge of the nail   _____

13. The nail plate is composed of a substance called:
    1) collagen   3) keratin
    2) melanin   4) cartilage   _____

14. The nail plate extends from the nail root to the:
    1) lunula   3) nail bed
    2) cuticle   4) free edge   _____

15. The reproductive organ of the nail is the:
    1) matrix   3) hyponychium
    2) lunula   4) eponychium   _____

16. The digital bones of the fingers are called:
    1) metatarsi   3) phalanges
    2) metacarpi   4) clavicles   _____

17. The palm of the hand consists of:
    1) 8 carpal bones   3) 10 phalanges
    2) 5 metacarpal bones   4) 6 dorsal bones   _____

18. The ulna is the large bone on the little finger side of the:
    1) wrist   3) upper arm
    2) hand   4) forearm   _____

19. The wrist bone is called the:
    1) carpus   3) digit
    2) metacarpus   4) radius   _____

20. The function of the extensor muscles is to:
    1) straighten the hand and   3) separate the fingers
       fingers
    2) close the hand and   4) rotate the wrist
       fingers   _____

21. The function of the flexor muscles is to:
    1) open the hand and   3) rotate the hand and
       fingers   fingers
    2) bend the wrist and   4) adduct the fingers
       fingers   _____

22. The ulnar nerve supplies the:
    1) thumb side of the arm   3) fingers
    2) little finger side of   4) wrist
       the arm   _____

23. The radial nerve supplies the:
    1) little finger side of   3) thumb side of the
       the arm   arm
    2) palm of the hand   4) wrist   _____

24. The ulnar artery supplies the:
    1) thumb side of the arm   3) back of the hand
    2) little finger side of   4) forearm
       the arm   _____

25. The radial artery supplies the:
    1) thumb side of the arm   3) palm of the hand
    2) little finger side of   4) back of the hand
       the arm   _____

26. Furrows in the nails may be caused by injury to the nail:
    1) epidermis   3) layer
    2) cells   4) matrix   _____

27. Before using any manicuring implement, it should be:
    1) wiped with tissue   3) cleansed and sanitized
    2) wiped with a towel   4) washed with soap and
                                  water   _____

28. Blue nails are usually a sign of:
    1) high blood pressure   3) poor blood circulation
    2) systemic illness   4) a lung disorder   _____

29. The common name for tinea unguium is:
    1) hangnails   3) ringworm of the nail
    2) ingrown nails   4) brittle nails   _____

30. Filing deep into nail corners may cause:
    1. blue nails   3) ingrown nails
    2) onychophyma   4) brittle nails   _____

31. Hangnails are caused by:
    1) thick lunula   3) thin matrix
    2) thin dermis   4) dry cuticles   _____

32. Split nails are often associated with what type of deficiency?
    1) dermal   3) systemic
    2) symptomatic   4) hormonal   _____

33. Nails having wavy ridges are polished with a slightly wet
    buffer over which is spread a small amount of:
    1) pumice powder   3) oil
    2) nail cream   4) clear polish   _____

34. Hangnails are caused by:
    1) infection   3) a nail deficiency
    2) neglect of nails   4) poor nutrition   _____

35. Splitting of the nail may be caused by filing:
    1) lightly   3) slowly
    2) rapidly   4) carelessly   _____

36. Hangnails are treated by softening the cuticle with:
    1) oil   3) pumice
    2) remover   4) strengthener   ____

37. Furrows in the nails may be caused by:
    1) allergy   3) a systemic condition
    2) dermatitis   4) a primary condition   ____

38. Splitting nails are often associated with extreme:
    1) oiliness   3) moisture
    2) dryness   4) cold   ____

39. Normal cuticle that forms around the nail is always:
    1) thin   3) smooth
    2) rough   4) thick   ____

40. An infected nail should be opened and treated by a:
    1) manicurist   3) pharmacist
    2) physician   4) cosmetologist   ____

41. Instruments sanitized with alcohol should be immersed in a
    70% solution for:
    1) 30 minutes   3) 20 minutes
    2) 15 minutes   4) 8 minutes   ____

42. To loosen the cuticle, use the following instrument:
    1) cuticle pusher   3) orangewood stick
    2) cuticle nippers   4) nail file   ____

43. A manicure should be given:
    1) once a month   3) every six weeks
    2) twice a week   4) once a week   ____

44. The purpose of buffing the nail before applying a sculptured
    nail is to:
    1) ensure greater adhesion 3) add color to the nail
    2) remove residue   4) add gloss to the nail ____

45. When mending with a nail wrap, file the split or chipped
    portion of the nail with a/an:
    1) emery board   3) nail file
    2) buffer   4) electric drill   ____

46. To smoth a nail wrap, use an orangewood stick dipped in:
    1) alcohol   3) polish remover
    2) disinfectant   4) cuticle remover   ____

47. Why is it important to sanitize a client's nails before applying
    sculptured nails?
    1) to ensure proper   3) to help prevent fungus
       adhesion   from forming
    2) to soften the nail   4) to dry the nail   ____

48. When applying a nail tip, buff the nail:
    1) where nail tip meets the free edge
    2) at the tip of the free edge
    3) in the corners of the nails
    4) just above the lunula ____

49. When affixing a press-on artificial nail, adhesive should be applied:
    1) to the center of the nail
    2) inside the artificial nail
    3) under the free edge of the nail
    4) on top of the artificial nail ____

50. During a nail dip, the nail should be inserted into an acrylic dipping powder for:
    1) 2 minutes
    2) 60 seconds
    3) 5 seconds
    4) 5 minutes ____

ANSWERS TO THE STATE BOARD EXAM REVIEW

1-1	2-2	3-2	4-2	5-4
6-3	7-1	8-3	9-2	10-3
11-1	12-2	13-3	14-4	15-1
16-3	17-2	18-4	19-1	20-1
21-2	22-2	23-3	24-2	25-1
26-4	27-3	28-3	29-3	30-3
31-4	32-3	33-1	34-2	35-4
36-1	37-3	38-2	39-3	40-2
41-3	42-3	43-4	44-1	45-1
46-3	47-3	48-1	49-2	50-3

HINTS ON HOW TO PASS YOUR
STATE BOARD EXAMS

These helpful hints have been prepared for your benefit. Read them carefully; they will assist you in passing the state board exams.

Personal Appearance

To present a good appearance and feel your best at the exam, use the following checklist as a reminder.

A. Personal Appearance
   1. Hands and Nails:
      - ☐ Hands clean and free from stains.
      - ☐ Nails clean and manicured.
   2. Hair:
      - ☐ Hair clean and properly styled.
   3. Face:
      - ☐ Face clean.
      - ☐ Proper facial makeup.
   4. Teeth:
      - ☐ Teeth clean and free from stains.
      - ☐ No dental defects.
   5. Offensive Odors:
      - ☐ No body odor.
      - ☐ No breath odor.
   6. Posture:
      - ☐ Correct standing posture.
      - ☐ Correct sitting posture.
      - ☐ Proper walking posture without shuffling feet.

B. Clothing Appearance
   1. Uniform and Regular Clothing:
      - ☐ Clean and pressed.
      - ☐ Hemline even.
      - ☐ Neat and properly fitted.
      - ☐ No slip showing.
      - ☐ Free from stale odors.
   2. Shoes and Hose:
      - ☐ Shoes properly fitted and heels straight.
      - ☐ Shoes shined.
      - ☐ Hose clean and free from runs.

Proper Mental Attitude

Adopting a calm, sensible attitude will help you overcome the nervousness often associated with the taking of an exam. Remember that exams are not given to make any students fail, but to do justice to all students. State board exams are given in order to find out what you know. If you have been studying and reviewing your textbook and notes, there is nothing to fear; the exams are graded fairly.

Being well rested will help you to function at top speed on the day of the test. Be sure to get sufficient sleep on the night before the exam. Try to avoid any hurry, worry or excitement before the exam.

Required Supplies

When taking an exam, you will need lead pencils, soft eraser, timepiece, required implements, admission card and other materials specified by the examiners.

Be on Time

Learn in advance how to reach the building where the exam will be held. Allow sufficient time for travel. Being on time for the exam will save you annoyance and delay.

Before the Exam

1. Go to your assigned room at once. Take your seat and be comfortable.

2. Make sure that you have all your required supplies.

3. Check timepiece for correct time. Note the time limits of the exam.

4. Listen carefully to the examiner's instructions and fill out all necessary forms as directed.

5. If the instructions are in printed form, read them over carefully and follow them exactly as indicated. If anything is not clear, ask the examiner.

6. Remember, do not sign your name on the exam paper unless told to do so by the examiner. If you have been assigned a number, place it in the proper place on the exam paper and answer sheet.

At the Written Examination

Be ready to start when the signal is given by the examiner.

1. See how many pages there are to the exam, how many parts it contains, how many test items are to be answered and whether all required answers or some are optional.

2. Watch your time and try to answer as many test items as possible within the time limit.

3. Read each test item carefully. Answer each one consecutively and place answers in proper spaces.

4. Do not spend too much time on any individual item. If you come across a difficult one, place a small check alongside it and return to it later.

5. If you are doubtful about any item, place a small question mark alongside it and return to it later.

6. As the exam draws to a close, allow a few minutes to answer those items which have been left blank.

7. If you finish before the time is up, review all answers, correct mistakes and answer doubtful items.

8. When you are finished, return the exam paper and answer sheet to the examiner.

Hints for Practical State Board Exam

1. Make sure that your hands are clean.

2. Wear a uniform that is spotless and pressed without wrinkles.

3. Use only clean and sanitized implements on model.

4. Observe sanitary rules during practical test.

RECOMMENDED READING LIST FOR FURTHER STUDY

Art of Nail Wrapping by Carol Cullen.
A comprehensive study of the techniques used in the art of nail wrapping to encourage the growth and strength of the real nail. Includes facts for beginners, repairs, transplants, helpful hints, straightening a hooked nail, correcting an inwardly curved nail, as well as nail fashions.

A Woman's Guide to Business and Social Success by Ruth Tolman.
This text includes all topics for success in the business world. It covers all facets of professional appearance, and features hand care as well as manicuring. This text will prove invaluable not only in developing your professional image, but will also reinforce your recommendations for your clients' image development.

Encyclopedia of Nail Beauty by Mary Elizabeth Norton.
As an encyclopedia, this provides you with 100 ways to grow longer and stronger fingernails. It contains an abundance of special tips that will expand your ability to correct nail problems and provide clients with useful guidance for the preservation of nail beauty between appointments.

Fingers and Toenails in Health and Disease by Dr. Herman Goodman
A special cosmetician's edition that outlines proper care of the nails and offers many suggestions for the prevention of disease. Includes a dictionary of abnormal nail conditions.

Hands by Linda Rose.
Hand language...what it reveals about you, about him...the mystique of our hands. The owner of the most photographed hands in the world tells how to care for, exercise and pamper your hands. There are tips to nail biters (how to stop) and practical advice to the woman whose hands are regularly exposed to water. This book has beautiful photographs, all keyed to help the reader on the road to healthier, lovelier hands.

Nail Techniques by Gloria Philips.
This complete and well-illustrated publication concerns the wide variety of nail treatments as well as advanced techniques of beautifying the nails. The book covers facts about nails, nail wrapping, manicures, mending, sculptured nails and nail tipping. The illustrations are complete and easy to follow. An excellent reference for all professionals.

Nail Technology by P.J. Hughes.
Learn the basics of manicuring along with the newest trends, styles and techniques in this full-color, step-by-step text. Wrapping, nail extensions, tools of the trade, nail art, nail anatomy and nail disorders are all covered—teaching up-to-the-minute style sense as well as professional skill.

Standard Textbook of Cosmetology by Constance V. Kibbe.
This completely revised edition features a new format, approximately 1,000 illustrations, and a detailed breakdown of basic plus up-to-the-minute subjects such as nail wrapping, chemical blow-outs, the metric system, acid and neutral permanent waving systems, and blow-styling. Each chapter sets forth the learning objectives and the easy reading style enhances learning and retention; making this text popular with both students and teachers. Suitable for professional-level training of cosmetologists, it considers the licensing requirements of every state.

The Professional Art of Nails by Linda J. Ware.
This book contains step-by-step procedures for creating beautiful sculptured nails and other types of artificial nails. It covers everything, from the table setup through shaping and sealing. Close-up black and white photographs accompany each step of the procedure, making this book easy to follow and a pleasure to use.